RUNNING
IN THE
MIDPACK

MARTIN YELLING AND ANJI ANDREWS

RUNNING IN THE MIDPACK

HOW TO BE A STRONG, SUCCESSFUL AND HAPPY RUNNER

BLOOMSBURY SPORT
LONDON • OXFORD • NEW YORK • NEW DELHI • SYDNEY

BLOOMSBURY SPORT
Bloomsbury Publishing Plc
50 Bedford Square, London, WC1B 3DP, UK
29 Earlsfort Terrace, Dublin 2, Ireland

A catalogue record for this book is available from the British Library

Library of Congress Cataloguing-in-Publication data has been applied for

ISBN: TPB: 978-1-4729-7340-5; ePub: 978-1-4729-7341-2; ePDF: 978-1-4729-7342-9

2 4 6 8 10 9 7 5 3 1

Typeset in Minion by Deanta Global Publishing Services, Chennai, India
Printed and bound in Great Britain by CPI Group (UK) Ltd, Croydon CR0 4YY

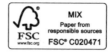

To find out more about our authors and books visit www.bloomsbury.com
and sign up for our newsletters

This book is dedicated with love to my Dad who never ran but always just got it. Everything I do is to make you proud, and I run with you always. – Anji

To Ruby, Sonny and Beau, run through life with patience, passion, courage, curiosity and love. – Martin

Contents

ONE

THE MIDPACK RUNNER

RUNNING IS FOR YOU

We love to run. We love that it pushes us, stretches us, asks us difficult questions, challenges us. We love that it also calms us, and gives us space, time just to be, but also time for others. We love the scope for striving and improvement, exploring faster, longer and getting stronger. We love the way running captures us – body, mind and spirit. We love how running connects us to people, places, nature and landscapes. We love its simplicity, but also its complexity.

We want this to be a book that nourishes your running, that helps you cultivate running progress and that brings even more joy to your running.

We run. We are runners.

Some of us have a physical activity conscience. We just feel it's something we have to do.

We run and we are the midpack. All of us. We're not defined by finish positions, split times, performance, miles run per week, segments chased, personal bests (PBs), number of race starts or race finishes, or DNFs (did not finish). Statistics are not what make us a runner. They sometimes motivate us, we use the numbers, but we don't identify ourselves by them.

The middle of the pack is no longer a place defined by finish times and percentages, and people in the middle of the pack can display just as much motivation and ambition (although with different goals) as those at the front.

Yes, running is something we do, but it's also something we *are*. Sometimes we identify as a runner alongside being a mother, a father, a daughter, a son, a teacher, an accountant, a grandparent, a bus driver, a manager, a writer, an electrician, a human. Running isn't everything we do, but it does shape who we are and how we interact and engage with the world around us.

We're real people and the midpack is a place where we hang out. It's sociable, but it can also be meditative. We run for the sake of it. We run for the challenge and for our goals. We simply love being outside.

We regularly move around in this midpack place we call home. The midpack has range. It's an environment where our running matters. Where we push ourselves, sometimes more than others, where we pull our fellow midpack along, but where we also rely on them, where we tackle demons, we face fears and we challenge perceptions. We're not the winners, but we're rarely right at the back, we're everywhere in between.

We wear big shorts, short shorts, we sometimes dribble, we have funny strides, dress like this, act like that, run like whatever, we couldn't really give a … . We care about each other, we care about you, we care about running companionship, we care about making and keeping friends, we care about being there, we care about showing up, we care about being on the line, we care about giving it what we've got on the day, we care about making the finish (most of the time!), however we can.

Oh, and we always know where the great coffee is afterwards.

We're past starting out. We've been at the back, we're rarely at the front but it's fun to try. We've done the beginner apps, the first-timer training plans,

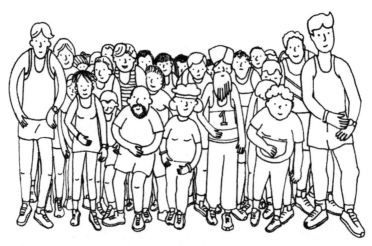

The midpack. Where everyone is at.

we've wrestled anxieties and race day nerves (we still do, they just feel a bit different). We've failed, we've tried again, and failed again. Sometimes our training works, sometimes it doesn't.

We're committed. We run regularly. It's not often that we totally lose our way with our running but it does ebb and flow. Even when many of our friends are runners, we still lose our desire-to-run mojo sometimes. Sure, we can all list our personal bests but our favourite stories are often about the times it all went wrong. We run in seasons. We have those months where our running just clicks and everything feels amazing, but we regularly have seasons where everything we do feels like an all-out, grind-out effort.

We are inspired by the people who are like us just as much as the pros. We say 'well done' to anyone who finishes, and we admire those who take prizes home, too. We are motivated by everyone who shows up.

For many of us, the only place we've ever been is the midpack. The midpack isn't a perfect place. It's full of possibilities. We like it there.

The midpack is our place, your place, and everyone else's.

RUNNING IN THE MIDPACK

It's through speaking and sharing ideas about running, expressing hopes and aspirations, worries, anxieties and concerns, reflections and reviews that coaching, progress, personal development and change take place.

Throughout this book, we'll explore backgrounds, contexts, expert thinking and opinion, scenarios and solutions concerning these, and take a peek at how runners live, thrive and move in the midpack. We will offer practical advice that you might want to experiment with, explore, think about or leave alone.

It's the movement that takes place in the middle of the pack that makes it a special place.

The midpack isn't a fixed place, and movement in the midpack isn't necessarily unidirectional. It's not always about relentlessly pressing forwards or sliding backwards. Instead, you can intentionally focus on ways to run in the midpack. You can opt to set the bar high, get your race face on and pull out all the stops towards progress, or you can take your foot off the gas, knock it into cruise control and be mellow. The midpack has many spaces along a continuum of people, aspirations, motivations. It's like finding your place on the wave in a surf break; we can't all be on the peak, sometimes we're waiting down the line, sometimes we're out the back, sometimes we're paddling through the break and occasionally we're washed up on the beach!

How you approach your midpack running depends on many, often shifting, motivations, aspirations, personal situations, contexts, challenges, risks and realities. We'll look at lots of these things, but what is clear to us – and therefore will represent a recurring and constant thread throughout the book – is the notion of *process*, and specifically, for us as midpackers, to be able to *trust the process* in our running.

Trusting the process means you know the highs and lows that come with training. It means you understand the value of your bad days as much as the good ones. You know how important rest is. You trust that it's not always going to be easy. Trusting the process means you are reflective about your running and that you (hopefully) arrive at your target race feeling prepared for and confident about what lies ahead. You know your race strategy and you trust that it will work, and there's no need to panic. You might have coaches, clubmates and friends you can lean on for support but when it comes to it, it all comes down to you.

We will explore how the process of getting your mind, your training, your nutrition and your race days right for you can help you to grow and nurture this trust.

THE THREE CLASSIC MIDPACK SPOTS

We're all different. In running parlance, some folk just choose their parents more carefully and have the genetic toolkit to gazelle about. For some, running just comes easy(er). With training, and with different types of training, runners also adapt differently. The stimulus applied (i.e. the type of running completed, the frequency, volume, intensity, duration, time, etc) and the motivations and aspirations sitting behind them, all add up to the fact that running and runners are not equal. What this means in reality is that the midpack is made up of many different types of runner at different points in their running journey.

It is relative; the swell of the midpack is a changing place. In some smaller, low-key events, races or parkruns, the midpack is you plus a few friends. In bigger events, the midpack could be hundreds of runners deep, and in large mass-participation races over longer distances, the midpack can stretch for miles and miles!

Moving in the midpack is as much about the hard-nosed realities of your fitness, your genetic disposition, your training status and your approach to training and racing as it is about the process of the softer side of your engagement with the midpack. The midpack is a state of mind as well as a physical space.

Running towards the pointy end of the midpack

This is when you want to give it full beans! Perhaps you've been targeting an event for a while and simply want to give your best effort on a given day. This happens when you are running with confidence. Your confidence might go up when you have been running fast with your club, and have been challenged within a group of friends and fellow midpackers. You might feel you're taking confidence from the process of training for a race, having a plan, ticking the sessions off along the way.

Confidence in racing comes from confidence in training. How to nurture, gather, harness and effectively maintain this confidence (and its related psychological friends and adversaries) will be explored in Chapter 2. At that sharp end, you feel relaxed and prepared, ready to put your foot down. Nervous energy for a targeted race seems to provoke this response as well. You have your splits in your head or programmed into your watch, and you know hitting up the front will allow you to get straight into that pace. It's a brilliant feeling to puff out your chest and stand tall at the front.

Being slap bang in the middle of the middle

This is often our favourite place to hang out. It's where the great conversation happens. It's safe here. We can push on if we're feeling it and we can be cautious here if we've got a niggle. The middle is great if you have a hangover, if you're tired, if you just made it to the start or you want to encourage your mates. This is the chill zone. We are comfortable here and we like it.

Ending up in the middle happens if you're being overly cautious sometimes, too. We look at our watches and think: 'Oh hell, this is too fast, I'm going to blow up, I need to back off' without giving our legs the chance to prove that they can achieve more.

Hanging at the back

Aren't those days of running slower than your average pace special sometimes? Hanging out at the back allows us the greatest social freedom in running. We are free to encourage everyone faster and slower than us, we aren't so out of breath that we miss out on catching up with a friend at our side. Hanging at the back allows us to be a pacer, a motivator and often just a very chilled-out version of ourselves. We can sometimes hang out at the back if we've got a bit complacent. Or a bit injured. Or we have been on a long old week of shift work. Being at the back isn't half as important as the fact you showed up when not everyone would.

FINDING YOURSELF IN THE MIDPACK AND THE REASONS YOU'RE THERE

Harmony in the midpack is created through aspirational contentment. It comes from managing the ebb and flow of the push in the midpack. Intentionally, we adopt an approach that purposefully doesn't strive for 'progress', 'more' or 'better'.

1. Racing

Sometimes you're in the midpack because you've got your game face on. It's race day. Racing gives you that goal, that 'something' you can aim for. Race day is what you've paid for in cash for your entry and a lot of sweat in your training. You got yourself to race day after dealing with whatever battles came along the way – it's unlikely you had none. You find yourself drawing on everything you have been practising in training, from every session you showed up for and every workout you felt like you nailed. Big races will often pen or corral you into predicted finish times but the chances are that without them you'd still be confident about where you should be. We think racing is so important in the midpack that we gave it its own chapter.

2. Socialising

Sometimes you're in the midpack because you're there with your friends. Being a regular runner, you will probably know a lot of other regular runners, it's often the best (or only) time you get to catch up. Running with your friends allows you to talk through things, listen and vent if you've had a crap day. Or week. It's the perfect time to rant or to rave. You're in the midpack because sometimes it kills two birds with one stone. It's a gloriously social activity that allows you to exercise at the same time. The social bit can be more important than the running bit, and we are cool with that.

3. Training status

Sometimes you're in the midpack because that's just where you are at. Your training status is defined by the running you've done, how many injuries you've had, how well you've been eating and the quality of your sleep. We'll look at training status and what affects it later in the book, but you've run in the midpack for long enough to know where you fit in. You know what should feel 'hard' and you don't always need your watch to tell you that. You belong in the midpack when you are improving, when things are going well. You belong in the midpack too when you are sliding backwards. You have gone through the process so many times that you know the midpack well enough to know which area within it is yours.

4. Head state

Sometimes you're in the midpack because it's where your head is at. You have been motivated. You haven't been motivated. You've had goals and you've had to let your goals slide at times too, and that's OK. Your head has been totally in the game or for ages it just feels like nothing has clicked. The more you run, the more you understand your body and what makes it break down, and hopefully that's the same for your head. We will get more into the deep psychology bit later in the book.

You will recognise that glow of confidence, usually after achieving a personal best (PB), which will make you want to run and run some more and just ride on that feeling for as long as you can. You're in the midpack when you have had a race written in your calendar that has been the focus for your running for a while. The process you've gone through to get there has kept you motivated and/or it's given you that beautiful 'fear' along the way. You get yourself to your goal race with your stomach like a washing machine, a bit like in your early days of starting out, because it means that much.

5. Ability

Sometimes you're in the midpack because of your ability. Look, let's face it, some runners chose their parents better than others and despite all the miles we might clock up, we're unlikely to be on the next plane out to the Olympic Games. There, sorry we broke it to you. We can all improve, some more than others, but inherited genetics have a part to play. 'Ability' seems like an odd word to use because of course you're able to run, and move, and train. You are able to enjoy your running and push yourself. You show up, you compete. You pin a race number on the same as everyone in front of you or behind you at the start. You can churn out results that some of your friends and colleagues might envy but you're not going to trouble those top finishers. You are in the midpack because that's where you belong. You aren't blessed with perfect running mechanics. You aren't paid to work on them, either. Being in the midpack means you just aren't as fast as the people at the front, for now, and that's OK.

It's great in the midpack and it's probably a lot less pressured than if you were someone who's expected to win every time, though once in a while you secretly wonder what that would be like.

6. Choice

Sometimes you're in the midpack through choice. You might have that deep underlying something, potential, whatever, but through choice in your running, in commitment, or life in general having better stuff for you to do, you have chosen to leave that potential where it is and you've never given what it takes to unlock it. You might not even know it's there. You're in the midpack because perhaps you've always gone through the same processes and you've enjoyed them so much you don't want to give any more. You are in the midpack because you've chosen to stay in it. You've made a conscious effort to not drop out of it. You've consistently kept running and there have been no gaps in your commitment that might have forced you to come back to running and start again.

You chose the midpack for racing, socialising, your training status, your head state and your ability.

SEASONS – MOVING UP, DOWN AND THROUGH THE MIDPACK

To make progress in running, whether that's a faster time or going further, you have to be prepared for the fact that it's going to hurt sometimes, so it's worth asking questions of yourself, such as: 'how much am I prepared for this to hurt?' and 'what am I afraid of?' To get faster, it's probably going to take that 'red-line' feeling where you rinse yourself at the threshold of discomfort and leave it all on the road for as long as you can. You have to trust that the process of going through this is worth it for meeting your goal. Whatever that goal is.

Running comes in seasons and it's helpful to look at it that way. Nothing lasts forever. Change and progress can be healthy. Where you are in the midpack happens for a variety of reasons, often unconnected to your running. We are going to look at that more when we talk about your foundations in Chapter 3 on whole body health.

You might be guilty of selling yourself short. How many conversations have you started at a race by immediately letting a person know you are injured/have been injured/probably have an injury brewing? You are sandbagging in case you run slower than you did last week, slower than you think this person might run. But are you also setting the bar low for yourself? While you should have some idea of your capabilities, you might be underselling yourself by having expectations that fall short. It's important to learn that balance.

Something we see a lot that holds people back in the midpack is not becoming comfortable with discomfort. We are often all too happy to coast along in our most comfy running slippers. Oh yes, you know the ones! Yet it's also about getting the balance right between allowing yourself to get into that uncomfortable state without doing too much too soon and getting injured. We are going to walk you through that careful, glorious balance that is the knife-edge between overloading and injury and show you how to get the most out of training with purpose in Chapter 4.

Comparison can be a good thing – shhhh, look at how you perform on a Strava segment if you know it's there! But a classic midpack mistake is to compare yourself a little too much to what others are doing rather than focusing on your own training process and trusting that it's right for you. You might also be comparing yourself to a different version of you from the past. We are going to look a lot at your identity and history in Chapter 2, so get ready to have those conversations with yourself. Comparison can be damaging to confidence and it's definitely something to be cautious of if it's making you move reluctantly backwards or step right out of the midpack.

We are also going to look a little at identity in Chapter 2, particularly how you see yourself as runner. If you aren't sure if being in the middle of the pack qualifies you as a 'real runner' (for what it's worth, we do and you are!), you might be making the mistake of cheating yourself out of proper, structured training, too. We are going to guide you through the importance of training, wherever in the pack you are, and hopefully you will see this is another way that will enable you to easily change your position in the pack.

We will get into whole body health in Chapter 3, starting at the very foundations of the most effective pillars for optimal health to enable you to be robust, prepared, strong and have longevity in your running, before moving into the nitty-gritty of training in Chapter 4. We are going to explore some technical bits of training without weighing you down with specific training plans or too much science. We hope to get you excited about approaching your training, planning your training, executing your training, changing things in your training, and reflecting on your training in order to help you reach whatever floats your running boat (we will help you to figure out what that might look like, too).

Chapter 5 explores the importance of nutrition for you, your running and racing, and we take a look at some of the tricky things you're going to have to work through, get comfortable with, explore, develop and refine so that you can run in the way you want.

Like all good journeys in running, we are going to finish with race day in Chapter 6. We'll look at how amazing racing can be, the practicalities you have to get right, and how to reflect on what happens in the days after the big day.

Nine ways you're in the midpack – 'yes, that's me, I do that!'

1. You actually like running. It's important (but not all-consuming) in your life.
2. You know what a wild wee is.
3. You have friends or a partner who runs (or at least who gets that you run!).
4. You have a physio/sports therapist on speed dial.
5. You regularly take part in timed running events where you prioritise social aspects as much as the run itself. 'Where is good for coffee?'
6. You prefer an early night to a party night before a race.
7. You have brilliant running stories to tell anyone who asks (or doesn't ask!).
8. You train. You train. You train.
9. You don't need to know the route inside out, as there's always someone to follow.

What's clear is that the midpack is a complex and loaded place. When you inhabit the midpack, your positioning and location within it is impacted by multiple, overlapping and complex variables influenced by fitness, training, race craft and strategy, psychology, motivation, confidence, nutrition and hydration, and the tricky blend of mixing this together to get it all right.

ON YOUR MARKS, SET, BANG! LET'S GO!

We'd love you to come on a journey with us in this book. At times, it might not work out how you expected, be about what you thought it would, or include what you want it to. We might not tell you what you want to hear, yet we hope we'll encourage some positive reflection. We'd like to raise a response, to even perhaps challenge some things you might think you already know and some established practices you've gotten too comfortable with. Always remember: we've got your best interests as a runner at heart. We want you to explore, trial and refine new, different, surprising, challenging, hidden and productive ways to move back and forth in the midpack and to understand why it's one hell of a place to live.

We believe you can run well in the midpack when you:

- have great self-awareness and when you know what makes you 'run tick';
- totally trust the process of your running;
- are truly content with the world of running you live in;
- are prepared to change, adapt, and learn to do running differently;
- smile; always have fun, be present in your running, be social, enjoy it.

And we want to show you how.

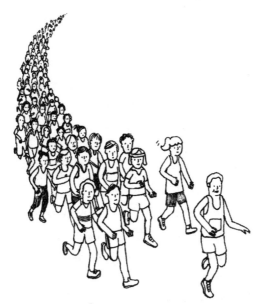

The midpack and I

THE MIDPACK AND I – FROM ANJI

I've been firmly embedded in midpack running since 2011. I grew up around competition as a competitive dancer but I certainly never excelled in PE at school – in fact I have so few memories of doing it, it feels like I barely took part. I went from doing occasional 5ks, to 10ks to half marathons and then became a club runner, quickly moving into leading groups and eventually coaching. My passion for running and shaping running for others – even if that just meant helping them to enjoy it – was a journey that took place rapidly over the course of a couple of years.

I started running in my late 20s and I loved that it didn't come easily (it still doesn't!). I got a lot of things wrong. I overtrained with very poor direction, I took great advice with a pinch of salt and in the early days, despite getting a few results I was really proud of, I broke down physically, seriously, frequently. Being a runner can break your heart at times but there's something about running that makes us in the midpack keep going back for more. Running is a beautiful thread that runs through our lives and we are fortunate to have it.

I was always an avid volunteer at running events, which led to me working for Events of the North, the race series run by Olympians Steve Cram and Allison Curbishley. I worked first-hand in mass-participation running event organisation, managed communications and built contacts through social media and coaching communities of runners who were mostly midpack runners like me. Working in this new world gave me a front row seat into racing that I had only ever seen from the other side, and it gave me opportunities to work with elite athletes whom I had long admired. The biggest takeaway for me was that they were always just like you and me. My passion for communication and community between runners led me to work, again first as a volunteer, on the 'Marathon Talk' podcast and then on to working with Martin. The 'Marathon Talk' community showed once again, and over and over, that runners are just the same deep down. I'm lucky enough to have been coached and mentored by Martin, who showed me how important process and reflection is to runners like me, as he guided me through the first marathon I'd done since receiving a heart condition diagnosis.

Like you, I have had the true pleasure of running with friends, channelling emotions into long runs to make sense of the hard times, harder days, bereavements. I have run in beautiful places I would have never otherwise seen, made friends with people I would have never otherwise have met, got close to what I have felt my physical limits were, met people who have changed my life, including my husband Paul at parkrun in 2014. We've crossed finish lines together and separately as I have coached him to distances and times I could only dream of. I've cried with joy, relief, disbelief that somehow it all just came together on the day. I have asked difficult questions of myself and I have challenged the thinking of those whom I have had the pleasure of coaching.

Running has been a huge part of my identity and has brought me more joy and great experiences than any other endeavour. This book explores not only the questions we are regularly asked as coaches, but also the bumps in the road we meet many times as a runner in the middle of the pack. What should be reassuring as you read is that we have shared experiences, dreams, passions, worries. We feel exactly the same on race day. We really care about getting the same things right, we wonder the same things about one another, find joy in the same experiences, ask the same questions of ourselves despite the very broad range of reasons why we do it.

Sure, running isn't everything. But in the midpack it's a massive part of us.

THE MIDPACK AND I – FROM MARTIN

There are some things, places, people and passions that are a constant reassuring, affirming presence in your life. For me, this has been running. As I approach 50 years of age, for the last 42 of those, running has been my constant companion, my critical friend, my saviour and yes, even sometimes my sworn enemy. I started running aged eight at primary school in Somerset. It offered stability, challenge, encouragement, it brought me praise, rewards, positivity, self-worth, it stirred in me ambition, stoked commitment, drive, motivation and tolerance, it taught me resilience, gave me the ability to overcome and endure, to face fears, to grow confidence and lastly, as running has grown with me, it's equipped and empowered me to share it with others. My 'running partner' has been a constant throughout life seasons, engaging with me, supporting me and challenging me in different ways at different times. Running has in so many ways been my life.

My sister was a double European cross-country champion, and a national champion with a 31-minute 10km (6.2-mile) personal best. My wife, Liz, is a two-time Olympic marathon runner with a 2 hour 28 minute PB, Commonwealth medallist, multiple National Champion and European and World cross-country medallist. I've competed internationally and participated in running events across the globe. In my early years of being a runner, it was all about doing everything I could to go faster, the pursuit of times, the learning how to train, the listening to my own coaches, British Milers Club stalwart Phil O'Dell, and in triathlon and duathlon Mark Booth. All of this while doing my PhD at Loughborough University and striving to keep up with the infamous George Gandy elite endurance group, listening to Alan Storey in his time as head of endurance at UK Athletics and Alec and Rosemary Stanton coaching Liz, all masters of their craft. It's been a privilege to experience the most pointy end of running. There's nothing quite like being on the start of the London Marathon in the elite tent (as a bag carrier for Liz I might add!) or in the call room of a major championships.

Running has taught me so much, as have runners. I love learning and, along with my friend Tom Williams (parkrun Global chief operating officer), we set up the UK's number one running podcast, 'Marathon Talk', back in 2010. Almost 10 million downloads later and we've been heard across the running world, yet significantly, we've also heard the stories of all runners. From Olympic and world champions through to first-time nervous marathoners, the intimacy, courage, surprises, challenges and incredible performances (and I don't necessarily mean 'fast' here) have continued to educate me about how running shapes and changes lives. Being involved with and seeing the rise of the parkrun movement has caused my passion for running for everyone to ignite. In my role as the coach for the London Marathon, I've guided thousands of runners to their first ever marathon finish. I've shaped and shared their training journeys, lived with them through the highs and lows of their running journeys, seen them progress up the midpack and slip right back down through it.

In this last decade, my own running has been spent largely living in the midpack, actually progressing comfortably back in that. I'll never go faster, I'll never run under 30 minutes for 10km (6.2 miles) again or finish in the top 10 of the National! But I'm OK with that. I'm OK with leaving running alone for a bit, with letting running serve me differently, with pushing when it feels right and with backing off when it doesn't. I can slip and slide in the midpack and enjoy every bit of the ride! I love seeing others progress in their own personal journeys – perhaps first coming at it with their lust for lost seconds or their passion to break barriers, but eventually realising the empowering ways in which being a midpack runner can transform, support and give so much to their lives.

So, here it is, in this book, for you.

T W O

PSYCHOLOGY

MESSING WITH YOUR HEAD

Running can be brilliant, but it can, if you let it, really mess with your head! Ever tipped up to a race and felt you didn't deserve your place on the start line? Ever talked your way out of a training session before you'd even started it? Ever been two-thirds of a way through a race, given up and beaten yourself up about it afterwards? Yeah, us too.

Our goal throughout this book is for you to continue to find ways to progress your running, nourish your running and find joy in your running. In this chapter, we want to help you see why things don't always go to plan, why you react the way you do, and what you can do about it to respond differently, better, to bring about a more desirable outcome next time around. Or simply to let it go and live with it without it getting you down.

This isn't a self-help book, and we don't believe in magic pills for this or quick remedies and fast fixes for that, but we do know that there are some games you'll play in your brain that really muck up your running potential, your running motivation, your running enjoyment and even your running friendships!

Dr Simon Marshall from Braveheart Coaching knows this well. It's Simon's day job to help athletes overcome fears and be braver to perform better. So, he's seen first-hand the struggles, tribulations, successes and failures that we all experience. Simon explains that: 'People are complicated. Despite running being really simple; technically it is just putting one foot in front of the other, when we put our muddled minds to it, we can unwittingly, unconsciously or sometimes even purposefully make it unnecessarily complicated.'

How you manage your headspace, how you mentally engage with your running training and racing and the world (both real and virtual) of running and runners around you can be a wonderful way to draw out the best of yourself and harness every bit of running potential and running love, but it can also be a dangerous, self-sabotaging, run-jeopardising, problematic and painful place to be when you get it wrong.

Getting it wrong is easily done, too. Often, you don't know, or don't see (or choose not to see) where things are not quite working out as you'd hoped, planned or intended. Before you know it, things you've been putting in place to 'help you and/or help your running' have sometimes subtly, and sometimes in quite an obvious way, assumed a destructive role.

You're not here to blame anyone, either. This chapter certainly isn't about getting all big and clever, being righteous, being judgemental about what you do 'wrong', do too much of, or too little of, it's not about making you feel small, or pointing the finger; rather, we hope we've learned a few things, made a ton of mistakes, helped others navigate through some running dilemmas and can share this knowledge so you can apply some of it to your context to give you some pointers to get back and stay on track. We certainly don't have all the answers and won't try to find fancy solutions for you.

We do want to explain and expose some of the pitfalls – the traps which are really easy to fall into when you're a runner. You know, the things you (in fact we all) do that are neither helpful nor productive, but you simply can't help yourself from doing sometimes. We propose some possible ways to work within, around and through these so that you can spend more time getting better, being better, doing your best more often and moving in the midpack however you want to.

Broadly speaking, things that mess with your running head can be categorised into three big groups:

1. Things about you – you know, all those things you worry about in relation to yourself, such as that you're not fit enough, you're too slow, you won't achieve your goals, you're anxious, fearful or worried, you'll let other people down, you're too fat, thin, weak or scared.

2. Things about other people – these are the things that aren't about you, but about others. Won't everyone be faster than you? Will you be last? Do you deserve your place on the line among all these other speedsters? What will they think of you?

3. Things about the big picture – this is all the wider area of racing, training, goal setting, defining success in certain terms, your end target, aspirations and satisfaction.

Of course, these three things are rarely, if ever, distinct from each other. They overlap, are inextricably linked, sometimes in complicated and confusing ways. They come and go when we least expect it, are influenced by the oddest and most surprising things, and sometimes can knock us off our running feet.

Arguably, it's not practical, possible or desirable to be the master of everything, all (in fact even any) of the time, and that's not what we're suggesting. But grappling with your running head, wrestling with some of the issues that trouble you, in and out of your running, can help you become not only a more effective, more successful, better (for you) runner, but also shift, shape and transform your life in many other significant ways.

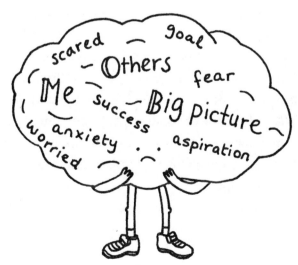

Things that mess with your running head

If we're not careful, running can get messy. Running can mean a struggle with some, all, elements of, or groups of these things some of the time, intermittently, in small doses, in big hits; it can be manageable, but sometimes also overwhelming and all-consuming. At times, it feels like we've got constant tricky dialogue with our wrestling naughty inner selves.

For Dr Simon Marshall, this is really relevant. Simon points to the 'gremlins in your head' that cause you to doubt yourself, to question your motivations, abilities, self-worth and personal value. This is all normal. Your job is to tackle this head-on and build strategies in your running, and in your life in general, that will turn these pesky gremlins into the voice of an angel that leaves you calmed, focused, confident and in control. But that is hard and is often about so much more than running. Although reflected by and mirrored in your running, the real issues, causes and concerns frequently sit much deeper.

We're far stronger and more capable than we've led ourselves to believe, and we need to give ourselves the chance, the opportunity and often the permission to jump into seeking ways to believe more is possible. Not more from our running (as that's the by-product) but more from ourselves. Get that complicated bit right and the running benefits will follow.

It's definitely complicated, though. Seemingly, these things that can mess with your head don't act in isolation. Often, they are inextricably linked together in complex and convoluted ways that are tricky, and sometimes hugely problematic, to disentangle, unravel or separate from previous life experiences. In so many situations, things that mess with your running head and can manifest in your running experiences are driven, influenced and impacted by things that sit way outside of running (and, most likely, way outside the remit of this book or the experience of the authors).

Yet, what we do know is that midpack runners happily invest in race entry, gear and training, but they don't always invest a great deal of time in their most powerful weapon: the mind.

We're going to take a gentle stroll through some of the major areas of head messiness, including:

- Confidence
- Perfectionism

- Emotions, anxiety and stress
- Motivation and mastery
- Self-esteem and judgement
- Social media pressures

All of these are things that you might experience in the midpack. We want to shed some light on how you can navigate and position yourself to be a content, confident and competent runner (however you'd like to be defined!).

CONFIDENCE – 'I'M JUST NOT GOOD ENOUGH'

We've all felt it and experienced it to some degree. We don't think there's a runner reading this who hasn't, at some point in their running career, had a confidence wobble, be it just a shiver of uncertainty about going for a run with a group for the first time or a full-blown trauma meltdown at a big race when you should be wearing your game face.

It's there all right, that internal voice that ramps up; it doesn't need much prompting, especially when a few triggers launch it at full volume. For all of us. 'I just don't know if I've got what it takes to do this.' 'Have I done enough training?' 'Am I up to it?' 'I'm just not good enough for this. I can't do it.' 'Will I let myself or others down?' 'These shorts rub, I hurt.' 'That's it, I'm done'.

Confidence is one of those tricky things in running that is shaped by many factors. You can't just 'be confident' and it's unlikely that you can be confident all the time about everything (hey Mr Perfect, I think they call that arrogance!). A little uncertainty when channelled in perspective can actually be a healthy aid to achieving desired outcomes. You've got to allow confidence to grow, to be shaped and nurtured through the uncertainty and threatening dilemmas that cause doubt and fear. It's a learned thing. It's contextual, personal, situational, specific, it ebbs and flows along a continuum, it's not always balanced. The trick is to understand your confidence boosters, know your confidence gaps, seek out your uncertainties and what triggers them, and work with this knowledge so you have control over the wobbles rather than allowing the wobbles to have control over you.

Confidence – the problem

Have you ever questioned your ability to do something? It's pretty certain that we all have. That time you pitched up to a big race you'd been training for and it all went south in the start area as you went through a crisis of confidence? Tears, fears and multiple trips to the toilet as a jibbering wreck cause your confidence to plummet and impact your ability to shine.

It's natural and normal to doubt yourself, things about you, and your running. Yet, if you practise and expose yourself to uncertainty, the uncomfortable can be quite transformative when you accept and work with it. Sport psychologist Dr Josie Perry explains: 'Confidence is when we trust our abilities, qualities and judgement to achieve what we have set out to do. Confidence boosts our levels of resilience and mental toughness so we can fully focus on executing our physical, psychological and perceptual skills.' She makes it sound so easy! Like it's this thing we can all effortlessly own. But it's riddled with complexity.

There are no quick-fix shortcuts to greater confidence. You can't take a supplement, get it in gel form, or pay a bit extra to buy 'The Best % Confidence Kit Booster' like you seemingly can with trainers, nutrition or fancy insoles. It's not kit. It's you.

Confidence is not only linked to your personal experiences as a runner, but also your life history and broader set of life experiences. We know this isn't easy to wade through and live with sometimes. In fact, for some people, running is *the thing* that they can press into and work on to help them discover fresh and hidden things about themselves that can shape and scaffold their whole inner being, and in doing so be wonderfully and positively transformative not just in their running but also in the wider world they inhabit.

Confidence in running (and everything else for that matter) is a delicate balancing act. It's linked to your identity, how you see yourself and get the best from yourself. It's about belief in process, execution of goals and balancing everything so that you don't tip the opposite way and become overconfident, self-assured or – dare we say it – cocky, leading you to make a mess of things just when you think you've got it cracked.

Being confident doesn't mean that you peacock around in your tiny shorts at the front of the start pen mouthing off about how fantastic you are going to be. Being confident in and about yourself and your running means you're happy and content to put yourself in situations that you find unsettling, uncomfortable, challenging or threatening and you recognise these situations as opportunities to learn and grow in your running rather than seeing them as times where the sky is going to fall down, your legs will drop off and it'll end in an unhappy running catastrophe for you.

Confidence allows you to crack on with a workout when it's getting tough. Confidence allows you to be comfortable running with people you've never run with before, no matter how fast or slow you perceive yourself or them to be. Confidence means you can roll up to an important race or event for you and be happy with your stage of readiness. Confidence helps you stick with a pacer in a race and it permits you to share your 'A goal' before a race without prefixing it with 'I haven't been training much lately because…'

Confidence – the fixes

It takes time and commitment to build confidence in running. There's not an immediate or straightforward pathway to follow that guarantees enhanced confidence in your running. You can't simply pull on some glittering new running kit or a fancy pair of trainers and feel your confidence soar (although it can sometimes help!).

Confidence is often quite specific to your running uncertainties and the things that you doubt about yourself, and that in turn cause you to question your running confidence. Yet there are things that you can build into your routine and life practice of being a runner that can shape and support your confidence and help you become more confident in your running.

We both really love the section in Dr Josie Perry's book *Performing Under Pressure* about sources of confidence. Josie talks about the importance of mastery, preparation, seeing others, self-talk, trust, the environment, social support, innate factors, the athletes' view, physiological state, self-presentation and competition to boost confidence. We're going to dig a little deeper into these now and reflect on how each could help you in your running to draw on and build some confidence.

Remember, it's really hard to do all of these things all of the time and some of them have some deep and complex layers. They certainly don't exist in isolation and they impact you and others in different ways and at different times.

Mastery

Confidence in running comes from confident preparation and training. You know when it's gone well and when it hasn't. When training has been producing good results, you've seen progress, you feel like you're on the road to mastering your game, your technique, your pace, your effort, your sessions. You've seen personal improvement, mastered the pace you're looking for and you've pinned down what's made you feel good before you get to race day. When you work towards a state of mastery, you relate well to the process of engaging in your running and through your striving for mastery you can draw confidence as your skill set to be a better runner develops. Spend gentle time enjoying the unhurried and gradual process of mastery. Confidence comes when you get it right. Learning and adaptation in running takes time. Embrace it and the ways in which you engage with it, and confidence will peak (for a more detailed look at mastery *see* p. 46).

Preparation

What constitutes 'effective preparation' means different things for different people. (There's much more about this in Chapter 4). Of course, this is normal! What determines appropriate and extensive preparation for you, in your world, depends on experience, commitment levels, aspirations, budget and available allowances.

Without doubt, however, great preparation breeds great confidence. Yes, preparation is about doing the hard yards, the miles in the bank, the workouts specific to your running goals, but confidence comes through getting prepped in more ways than that. It's also all the practical preparation that surrounds your running. This is both in your training and also racing. If you feel prepared, beyond the physicality of your training programme and towards broader aspects of your running goals in training and racing – such as nutrition, kit requirements, organisational and practical things like looking over the route the night before, working out how you'll get to the race venue, knowing what your stomach can cope with for race-day breakfast – then your confidence around your running performance improves.

Seeing others and vicarious confidence

This sounds a bit like 'vicious' confidence, which would be cocky. It isn't that. Instead, sometimes as a runner you think it's just you that is like you. That it's much easier for other people. That no one else experiences running like you. They are so much better cut out for this running lark than you are. The thing is, they are not, and often they are just like you.

When you see someone you perceive as 'just like you' doing something and think: 'I could do that', or at least: 'I think I could try and do that', that's vicarious confidence right there, and it rubs off on you. Taking cues from other people should be easy, but we know it isn't always and often there are many complicated barriers to work around and overcome. You can't take inspiration from others if you stay in the car frightened about joining that running group for the first time and don't put yourself in a situation that might surprise you. Look around at parkrun, or at your next training session, the next running event you carry bags at, spectate at, watch on the TV. The people there are – in some ways – just like you. It might not be obvious at first but when you look closely, you'll be able to take some serious inspiration and encouragement from others. What's more, it won't be long until you'll be the inspiration and confidence booster for other people.

Self-talk and verbal persuasion

This is otherwise known as praise and encouragement! When done well, it boosts your self-worth and primes your self-esteem, it helps you value yourself, your effort and your abilities and can be a real enabler to better confidence. Having someone believe in you, to hear them articulate that belief in a meaningful, genuine and authentic (even if sometimes surprising) way, can really help your confidence to grow.

Sometimes (potentially a lot of the time!), with low confidence you doubt your running ability, it just doesn't seem possible, doable, practical or achievable. However, when other people believe in you and when they tell you that you can do it, when they have more faith in your capacity and in your ability than you do, it helps you believe it's possible. Verbal persuasion from significant others done in an authentic way and, even more meaningfully, at the right time and in the right way for you, is an amazing confidence-affirming gift. A little gentle verbal pick-you-up can help impact and improve your confidence even when you feel your mind, body and legs are going to pieces.

Do you ever truly reflect or draw on verbal persuasion effectively? It's really easy to gloss over someone's encouragement and praise, perhaps because of your own embarrassment, self-doubt or fear. Think about the positive and encouraging things your friends and family say about your running (go on, there must be some!). Do you ever truly acknowledge these, take them on board, listen and hear them with intent, or do you idly cast them aside as a throwaway attempt at making you feel better? Notice, collect and remember these comments from people and add them to your armoury of positive reinforcement, praise and encouragement that you can carry with you as you run.

Trust

Running is and should be a really relational activity that allows you to connect with other people, feel empowered and have a sense of belonging. If you let it, and you want it to, it's great for making and maintaining positive, healthy relationships. Effective relationships in and around your running really matter when it comes to helping your confidence and trusting your key advisors, those that guide, shape and support your running self, all of which impacts your self-worth and confidence as a runner. Positive running relationships can come from running friends, running partners, family, athletics coaches, doctors, physiotherapists and even (!) your non-running friends. Good peer relationships matter as much as good coaching relationships – especially if you trust that they all have your best interests at heart. Sometimes this can feel contradictory (especially for the perfectionists among you) but learning to establish and maintain trusted running relationships, learning to listen to 'advice' (in the many forms that can take) and, importantly, faithfully acting on that advice, shapes you as a confident runner.

The environment

Exposure (or lack of) to your environment or surroundings can influence your running confidence. If you're not used to or don't know a place, route, terrain or surface well, then this can impact your running confidence. You don't become a different runner when you run somewhere new or different, despite your perception of your own ability shifting. For example, runners who spend all of their running time pounding the pavement can experience lower confidence when they first hit the trails or go off-road. This could be because of uncertainty in their ability, proprioception, worry over risk of injury, falling over or getting lost. How often do we runners hear 'hills, I can't run up hills'? This is more to do with insecurity, lack of confidence and misperception of ability to control and regulate uphill running as a result of lack of exposure to hill running. If you want to boost environmental confidence, do more of what dents your confidence and causes you to have confidence wobbles. With specific exposure comes reduced fear and anxiety and greater confidence. Confidence and security in running environments is when you feel that 'I love running here' feeling. If you have already run somewhere or you find yourself in surroundings you prefer, or feel more competent in, you're probably going to feel more comfortable. You're never going to feel as confident running on a surface you've never run on before as you do when you're taking in a course you've done 100 times before. Changes to your environment challenge your comfort, so you need to improve your confidence by getting uncomfortable more often in training.

Innate factors

This can be feeling like you have a natural ability, gift or talent, or its opposite, which is not feeling like a runner because of negative previous experiences, misconceptions about yourself or misperceptions about other people. You just need to accept that there are bits of you that are just 'you' and that's OK. Some people chose their running parents better and got the running gene that you didn't. Hey, that's perfectly alright, for them and you. Instead of worrying about a weird thing your arm does when you're running, or wishing your legs were just a little bit longer – or shorter – think about the things you've always been effortlessly good at. You might be a superb sprint finisher, king of a hill or have a superb flowing running style that people always remark upon. Focusing on these innate factors makes you feel confident. Give yourself one or two reminders of those things next time you're starting to struggle.

The athletes' view

Runners like to feel things are going our way. There's nothing better than simply knowing, the internal feeling backed up by external outputs, that you're on a roll! When your view of your running world is overwhelmingly positive, your confidence to run and in your running seems unbreakable. Training has gone to plan, everything is clicking, when the hammer is down you're cruising, with another gear to give, you're on a wave of good sessions, great results and positivity all round. When your world view of your running is on a high, unsurprisingly, your confidence is unshakeable. That peak state, however, is variable, largely not sustainable and almost always about to end! It's therefore better to become more content, settled, patient and secure with areas of running confidence that trouble you. It doesn't have to be right all the time for your running to be going right. One poor or below par run doesn't make you a crap runner. It's not true that 'you're only as good as your last run'. It takes many different runs to understand you as a runner – great, good and epic fail. Embracing your view of your fragility, running vulnerabilities and confidence shakers – and working with, around and through these, rather than against them by allowing them to take over or dominate your running self-view, is the way to a more rounded, better-grounded, stable, secure and happier runner!

Self-presentation

Feeling good about the way we look, how our body looks, even how we stand, can impact our confidence. Ever bought yourself a new pair of running kicks and when you pull those bad boys on you suddenly feel supersonic and like your 10k PB is about to get crushed? You're not actually faster, stronger or fitter, you're just presenting as such.

Some people feel more confident in a great pair of trainers; they have lucky socks, success pants or glory haircuts (we even know someone who has the same, dependable pins that they use for every race) or have a greater sense of belonging when they wear their club vest or milestone T-shirt. Think about what you do or could do when it comes to your physical presentation and if there are any tweaks you can make to shape it to present to yourself and the wider world your run confidence. (Tip, don't peacock in tiny shorts, it's not a good look!).

Competition

Competition is healthy. Putting yourself in competition where you feel comfortable to push, to stretch, to fail, to get it wrong, but also to get it really right, is vital in moving through the midpack. How you respond to that competition is what gives you the confidence edge. Competition should be your confidence teacher. You can learn great humility, respect, dignity, trust and courage through appropriate and relevant competition. Now, we're not saying pitch yourself up against sub 2-hour marathon runner and world record holder Eliud Kipchoge, just that developing a keen sense of competition with yourself and those around you can be a confidence booster rather than a confidence kicker – when you get your response right. Confidence through competition isn't just about 'beating X, Y, Z', or about taking joy in others' 'failure', or overinflated exuberance in your own success. Even when 'losing', you can still see gains through watching someone you identify as being 'the same as you' doing something you know you can do too. Just not yet.

Finally, fake it

Yes, we were surprised by this one too but wanted to add it to the list. That's right, you can get more confident by faking it. Sports psychologist and thought leader in emotions in sport Professor Andy Lane from the University of Wolverhampton says: 'Some people have a lot of ability but little confidence. Faking it helps them get to the start line, then when they get going and find that they are doing well, they gain confidence.' Acting with confidence is a well-learned emotion regulation strategy.

Five things confident runners say

1. 'I'm happy with where I'm at and ready to do my best.'
2. 'I feel good about myself and my ability to perform how I'd like.'
3. 'I am so loving my running right now.'
4. 'I've got this (and I know what to do to keep it that way).'
5. 'I'm focused on me, this race, right now.'

PERFECTIONISM – 'I'M JUST NOT HAPPY UNLESS IT'S RIGHT'

Have you ever felt frustrated that a run didn't go quite to plan (only 'most of the time' you cry!) and that it didn't work out as you'd hoped? Three classic scenarios in the midpack are:

- 'I didn't run as fast as I wanted to. Those lost minutes and seconds are going to ruin my day.'
- 'I didn't run as far as I planned today. My plan said 5 miles (8km) and I ran out of time after 3 miles (4.8km)/I gave up after 4 miles (6.4km)/I sacked it off feeling too tired at 2 miles (3.2km).'
- 'I got dropped! I was running with a pack, then they left me behind in a gear shift I couldn't handle.'

Usually, midpack runners feel that they've failed if their run wasn't fast enough, far enough, they felt terrible, they got dropped, or they just gave up. So why was that? How did you set that run up? How did you frame for yourself what success in that run was going to look like? Who set those expectations and why were they there in the first place? This is getting deep! But it's important.

If we're able to understand our feelings, to relate to them, to be curious about why we feel that way, to explore what history, experiences, behaviours and exposures have shaped us to think, feel and act in particular ways then we are more likely to be able to shift the dial in terms of those thoughts, feelings and actions and position ourselves differently.

This counts for our running, too. When we react in a certain way, such as placing an unreasonable amount of pressure on ourselves, getting frustrated, disappointed, or overanxious, or when we set ourselves unrealistic standards, it helps to take a step back from these behaviours. By noticing and assessing them (sometimes with help) we can explore if they are productive or destructive to the kind of runner we are, or want to be. Then we can put in place (again, sometimes with help) strategies to navigate us towards better running, whatever 'better' looks like for us.

We're going to look at some of these issues in turn and explore how giving them meaning in our own running can help us position our own running performance where we'd like it to be.

Perfectionism – the problem

Since when was running flawless, anyway?

Being automatically self-critical and piling massive pressure on yourself doesn't sound like a very happy, fun or healthy way to be in life generally, or in running. You like things to go well, we get that, everyone does. But we want you to explore whether striving for perfectionism is doing you more harm than good.

Professor Andy Lane defines perfectionism as: 'a personality trait that is characterized by a person's striving for flawlessness and setting high performance standards, accompanied by critical self-evaluations and concerns regarding others' evaluations.' Wow, on reading this, none of it sounds especially healthy or positive. Nevertheless, we are sure it resonates with you because it did with us.

When something is important to us we place emphasis on it, we pursue it with passion, rigour and intensity. For us in the midpack, obviously that's running, but it might go deeper as we find ourselves working towards a target event, race or time. Performance coach and author Steve Magness has written a lot about this with coach and writer Brad Stulberg including in the

2019 book *The Passion Paradox: A Guide to Going All In, Finding Success, and Discovering the Benefits of an Unbalanced Life*, which is one of our favourites. They keenly observe that there are times when this passion can certainly become destructive. When we set super-high performance standards (we don't mean running a new marathon world record but something relevant to you) we can get highly critical, disappointed, frustrated and overly harsh with ourselves when we fall short, which we inevitably will do. We should recognise instead that this doesn't define us as a runner or human being but should inform us as a learner and inspire us to be kinder to ourselves, be more appropriate with our aspirations and learn contentment as a response. This requires us to reflect on the process of working towards goals and aspirations regularly.

A key part of the definition of perfectionism is the notion that you strive for flawlessness and set very high standards; those two points alone can struggle to sit well together. It might be possible to achieve a flawless performance if you set the bar low for yourself, for example a runner with a mile PB of 7 minutes going to a race with a goal of hitting 8 minutes for the mile. A perfectionist would instead set the target of a 'perfect' inflexible and often very specific goal (those seconds matter, right?!) that forced them to work much harder. It's that inflexibility that causes the main issue.

Perfectionism also has a social side: thoughts and criticisms and beliefs about what other people are thinking. Perfectionists believe (notice that is this is rarely the reality, rather just the perfectionists' perception) that others are expecting that unless a high standard of performance is attained, then the person's worth will be reduced. How ridiculous does that sound when you read it back to yourself? Your worth as a human is reduced if you fail to realise certain (mostly self-set) standards as a runner? As coaches, friends and fellow humans, we don't think so. But it's serious. When your view of the world is clouded by the mistaken belief that how others see you is related to your running success it can set off and compound a string of complex anxiety and emotional issues both in and out of your running world.

The idea that respect from others is dependent on how well you run can become very negative and unrealistic. If the standard of performance set as a goal is high, often not attainable, and the belief that it must be attained is held, then things can get a little miserable. As an example: you're running a half marathon, you've diligently trained, you're in good shape, a bit uncertain (but hey, that's normal!), but you are driven to break that darn 2-hour mark (since you missed it by 10 seconds and then 23 seconds on the last two attempts!) and score your PB, so you've set yourself a pretty tight pace timeline. When you start to run, the miles clock by and you somewhat obsessively keep checking your GPS split every 400m, and despite hitting it in the early miles, as the distance progresses you slip further behind the pace standard you set and begin to become highly self-critical (because you are not running fast enough and somehow should find more effort, you're lagging behind, your goal has gone) and you believe other people are judging you negatively. This mindset while running is destructive, negative and certainly unpleasant. Anji personally experienced this more than once during her pursuit of a very specific and probably arbitrary half marathon PB and had a few miserable race experiences despite taking part in events she'd always wanted to do that should have been filled with joy from beginning to end. Luckily, though, you've got the power to turn it around and tackle your drive for your perfect run.

It's really important to note here that we do not believe you are defined as a human being by the time you run for a marathon (or 10k, or whatever for that matter!). If you're reading this and notice a few perfectionist qualities that resonate then it's relevant and important for you to know this.

Where do these perfectionist beliefs come from? Professor Andy Lane says they begin partly from your innate personality traits: 'Some people are highly motivated. To set an extremely challenging goal and expect a flawless performance you need high levels of internal motivation.'

Often, we see that runners who display high levels of perfectionism are also the individuals who have a strong need to achieve, but also that it can be people with a high fear of failure. Failure for a perfectionist can occur even when the performance looks good to the outside world. A runner who achieves a PB, but does not achieve their goal, for example with marathon times around the hour (sub 4, sub 3) might still consider this a 'failed' performance. No personality traits can be easily changed, so if you feel that you have perfectionist traits (note that perfectionism doesn't apply exclusively to sport; it will affect other areas of your life, too) then acknowledging them is useful.

It might not be possible to change your personality (nor do we want you to!) but you *can* change your reaction to events. That's where your power lies.

Environmental factors are important when it comes to perfectionism. Often, when we run with others, we begin to compare ourselves to those runners, or even to a former version of our younger, fitter, snappier self. This is normal and it's just how humans are wired. Nevertheless, the environment in which we run can lead to those negative perfectionists' thoughts when the standard of performance expected is overly high and runners are not encouraged to have plans outside of the time or position goal.

Instead, it is preferable to set *process* goals, which are not dependent on other runners, and focus on running smoothly and being relaxed, on being the best version of you at the time. Setting process-focused outcomes and in doing so being present in the now (the present moment) and how (the action steps planned/taken) is beneficial. If you recognise some perfectionist qualities in yourself, this can be hard to achieve but is truly transformational when you manage it. Learning to focus on what is going on in the here and now – what you are doing, how it feels, how hard or easy it is, the skills being used and noticing and reflecting on those that are absent – is a good strategy to manage the inner perfectionist. Remove the outcome; focus on the process.

Perfectionism can be a helpful friend but can also be a destructive foe. Perfectionism becomes destructive when you get into a circle of high expectations, negative emotions, negative self-talk, a sense of failure and low self-esteem. Perfectionists can postpone tasks rather than entering the cycle of training, or engage in self-depreciation, possibly to get positive support from others, and can push too hard, lack flexibility, exert too much control, and develop unhealthy, obsessive behaviours. It's not always productive to 'be the best you can be', especially when it's at any cost. In fact, stepping off the gas, taking stock, letting go, being satisfied, content and gentler on yourself can be equally 'productive and effective' – just differently.

We'd both say that we are working on ways to 'dampen' our perfectionist tendencies. Martin notices ambitious, performance-focused perfectionist qualities that have driven him to aspire to accomplishment throughout his life, whether that is striving to complete a PhD, be an international runner, win national championships, build a successful business or charity, or write a book (!). Anji has always been self-motivated and felt driven to go and get things for herself, feeling guilty when she relied on others, especially when building her self-employment. She is often guilty of setting specific perfectionist targets in running and definitely recognises herself in the section above about negative self-talk. We understand perfectionism drives us both in different ways but we see it can also be destructive and harmful if we are left to race relentlessly forwards without careful nurturing, clear orientation and supportive environments.

Perfectionism – fix it

Perfectionism doesn't have to be destructive. Giving yourself flexible targets that create healthy behaviours and goals you can achieve – and be happy with – is a key positive behaviour. Nail down that positive self-talk, and most of all learn to recognise when the opposite is causing you to self-sabotage. You can fix this!

Recognise it

You might not have ever thought of yourself as a perfectionist before. Anji, with her messy office, tendency to leave things unfinished and average-at-best race performances certainly never saw herself as striving for perfection until we started getting into this. But framing those race experiences as situations in which she was in pursuit of something tough and that ultimately spiralled into negative self-talk certainly resonated. A good starting point is to recognise whether or not you are doing any of these 'perfectionist runner' things and noting down where they are impacting negatively to your life in the midpack. Generating meaningful (we don't mean destructive or overly critical) self-awareness and noticing traits and characteristics in scenarios where you have reduced flexibility and strive for completeness, perfection and constant high standards in your running is a good start. How do you feel when you miss a day's training in your well-planned-out schedule? How do you feel when you don't hit that target time you had in mind?

Trust the process

Dig deeper into how. Realistically, running isn't going to be brilliant all the time. It's great if you can start seeking, discovering and finding joy in the process of running – whether that's your easy runs, runs with friends, workout sessions or races – even when you're not hitting a time, a distance you planned or being able to keep up with someone. Seeking joy in the process of running rather than always looking for outcome can make you happier and more content with your running even when it's not what you'd planned. When you do something in and with your running that you enjoy, when that makes you feel fulfilled, gives you purpose, brings some meaning to your life, creates social and relational connection, then you've got the balance right, because these are processes to embrace, cultivate and value over and above seconds in your running.

Relax FFS

Putting yourself under constant stress and worry is going to make you miserable. Cut yourself some slack, relax, understand that you're rarely going to get the best out of yourself by always being hard on yourself. Being kind to yourself is really important. Learn to let go of the itsy-bitsy things that growl at you when that run didn't work out. It's OK. You can choose to respond differently and do it differently next time.

Create the right climate in which to thrive

Understand what motivates you, what helps you flourish and learn to find ways to cultivate running climates that are enabling and powerful for you. What empowers you? Look back to the section on confidence and pick out what positively influences you. Keep any negative self-talk in check. One of Anji's coaches reminds her before most races and workouts that it's OK to have negative thoughts sometimes, it's just not OK to always act on them. Understand that goals are just that, and they won't always click, and that's fine, too.

ANXIETY AND STRESS

We're going to talk more about specific, trotting-to-a-Portaloo-20-times race day nerves in Chapter 6. Things that make you nervous or anxious can crop up every day, well before race day approaches. This is not about general anxiety disorder or a medical condition that may disrupt your head on a daily basis, but the nerves and doubts that might crop up and cloud your brain when it comes to just getting out there and getting running.

Anxieties for the midpack runner might take the shape of overthinking a niggle ('what if my calf pops again?'), presuming something is going to go wrong ('I can't do cross country, I might fall over') and often the fear of getting out of the comfort zone and running in a way that hurts. It's not always easy to get comfortable with being uncomfortable and many of you in the midpack will know if you're honest with yourself whether or not you avoid working hard in your running. Some of you will also worry about things over which you have no control. 'What if it rains?' 'What if it's windy when I go out? It's hard running into the wind.'

Before you know it, you've catastrophised the joy out of the whole process. This is where emotion regulation comes in.

Emotion regulation

Emotion regulation is not as simple as telling ourselves to 'keep emotions in check', nor is it maintaining a stiff upper lip and keeping emotions under wraps. We are all emotional beings and we all have the same breadth of emotions that we express or contain on a day-to-day basis. You might not cry at the drop of a hat but it's OK if you do at a finish line that means a lot to you.

Emotions are always there. There are the nice fluffy ones, such as starting a run feeling happy and energetic, and the unpleasant, but arguably helpful and necessary ones, such as experiencing anger, anxiety or misery. Emotions have the power to make us feel confident, tall, strong and fast but by contrast they can also leave us feeling sluggish, drained, like we can't move. Professor Andy Lane explains: 'Emotions have an evolutionary function; sometimes we needed to be energised, to fight off other people, animals, and at other times we needed to conserve our energy, possibly hide, when the risk of death was high.' In light of this, we can't just turn them off.

Now, we realise getting your workout done isn't exactly the same as hunting for food – or maybe it is in some ways – and finishing a race isn't quite the same as risking death (hopefully). Instead, running is connected to your emotions via the goals you set for yourself. We like to get into the best possible mindset, we feel good when we 'think positive' and depending on how successful our performance is, we experience positive or negative emotions. Emotions are really powerful and so having an awareness of them and building and shaping your ability to control, express and regulate them is a good thing. Incidentally, we don't mean suppress your running emotions here. If your running allows you to experience emotion (and we're sure it probably does, from elation to disappointment, and from pleasure to pain) then noticing these emotions – how you feel when they arrive, how you respond to them, what you subsequently do in your action and behaviour – is an important element of growing as runner in the midpack. This will help you learn regulation skills and strategies that will enable you to cope with everything running (and everything else!) can throw at you. It might even help you see an opportunity to use these skills in contexts and situations outside of your running where similar emotions emerge and you can respond appropriately.

How you might feel after a race

Positive
You're feeling sociable, you want to stick around and chat. You're wondering what you can do next, what's the next event you want to go for. You can't wait to tell someone what you just achieved. You're smiling, you're happy and it's obvious.

Negative
You'd rather nobody spoke to you and you just want to leave. You feel embarrassed because you missed a target. You look miserable and you don't want to discuss the race with anyone.

Nerves and anxiety in running and racing can be a good thing. We are going to get into that in Chapter 6 in more depth when we look at channelling them into good performance. Nerves show you care. Anxiety recognises that competition can feel threatening and gets you ready to spring into action. Feeling anxious presents itself in many ways you might recognise – are you a shoelace checker or a number repinner? Actions like these may actually be a good use of your nerves; a lace coming undone or a flappy race bib would definitely affect your run. You will know of runners who bounce up and down on the spot, others who stand very still and stare at the floor; both are probably experiencing exactly the same emotions and expressing them in different ways. We don't want you to become a robot. We're not telling you to stop feeling things, or to ignore how you feel, but we hope there are a few ways we can show you how to recognise emotions and regulate them through the process of training.

It takes practice, but it can be simply about reducing the intensity of the emotions you are feeling. How many times have you gone off too hard at the start of a race because you've built up so much anxiety while you've waited for the start signal to go? This is a great way to ensure you'll detonate in the later miles – and you know that from experience if it's happened to you before.

Some midpack runners get anxious about running hard and it leads them to really closely monitor how they are feeling, especially when fatigue sets in. This is not good. Professor Andy Lane explains that: 'If you are tired and anxious at the same time, anxiety intensifies how tired you feel, it leads to thoughts of not being able to cope, convinces you to slow down or stop.'

Flip that around for a moment and look at experienced elite runners, the pure racing snakes. They experience the same feelings as us. They are tired, they are uncomfortable, they are hurting, they are wondering if they have the capacity to carry on. The difference is that they have learned to use a workable toolkit to cope with it. They're likely to be able to accept that getting tired is part of the journey, and overcoming fatigue is part of the achievement. Pure racing snakes tend to accept and embrace fatigue rather than stress about it and then just crack on with their running. To us in the midpack, they probably look like they are coping much better than we are, and in a way they are, but it is their ability to regulate their anxieties that allows them to do so. That said, elites, like the rest of us, can and do have real issues around their emotion regulation at times. That's OK. This stuff is important to us as humans.

Emotion regulation – do your thing!

Getting emotion regulation right can have a powerful effect on your running. You can still feel anxious at the start of your race but you can recognise it as excitement and stay calm. Anxiety is simply there to tell you that the event is important, and you feel calm because you trust the process of the training you have done to execute your race plan like a boss. Hurting as you run towards a PB can be hugely motivational, it's when it's hurting and it's going wrong that the spiral can start.

You will be able to recognise deployment of effective emotion regulation strategies when someone comes to pass you in a race. The unregulated version of your response probably brings a wave of annoyance or anger and the unregulated you probably tries to respond by speeding up. With careful emotion regulation, however, you will find it easier to stay calm, trust the process that got you here and allow yourself to stick to your strategy rather than wishing bad things on the person who passed you. Just because someone else put a big effort in, doesn't mean your plan has to go out of the window. Faster runners will go past you, and that's OK. Emotion regulation means you might be able to instead use them as a marker, someone to keep in view while you stick with your plan rather than hunting them down at a pace that's outside your ability. Professor Andy Lane explains: 'Managing your emotions [that are caused] by how other runners perform is a good example of effective emotion regulation.'

Emotion regulation: fix it

You're not a robot

All of your emotions are valid, and they are OK. Don't try to ignore or squash them. Recognise them and accept who you are and what you're feeling. Monitor your feelings, they are part of the process.

Accept where you need to regulate your emotions

Anything that's having a destructive effect needs to be kept in check and worked on.

Make the change

Acceptance is the first step for all of this. Don't squash anything, but work out what you can change. Rely on the advice of others when you need to, look for and adopt strategies that you can mirror to keep yourself in check.

GOAL ORIENTATION, BEING MOTIVATED, AND WHY THEY LINK

We are a mixed community with very different goals, united by running in the midpack.

Some people in the midpack see goal setting and motivation as two separate things, but what we think is that they are, or have to be, intrinsically linked. The aimless wafting of easy, irregular, unscheduled running that goes on when you don't have a target race coming up proves that. There is of course a healthy place for aimless wafting (when you run because you just feel like it rather than because it's planned or you are driven to do so) but the chances are that it isn't going to get you ready for your A race (*see* p. 88), during which you'll run your best time. We're going to look more at how having a goal can shape your training in Chapter 4.

Goal setting can help you do stuff

Having a goal shapes what you do, what you plan to do, and gives you a bucket load of motivation. A goal is like a deadline you get at work, but in running.

Setting a goal might start with 'I just want to finish' and work deeper into a series of whys and whats, before you work on the when. Let's get deep with why we are doing it. We want to inspire someone, we want to be a good role model to our children, we want to raise money for a charity that's important to us. We want to go further because we can.

Golden goal setting rules

Be realistic
You need to have a real understanding of yourself and the constraints in which you work. Be realistic about what you're really capable of. It's OK for your goal to feel a bit distant, a little out there, out of reach yet visible.

Be flexible
Roll with all the ups and downs and build flexibility and fluidity within. Lacking flexibility, especially when you end up having to miss a run, means a goal and a plan is more likely to go out of the window.

Make it personal
Don't be overly influenced by other people! Your goals have to be all about you.

Be specific
Make it tangible, such as a goal finish time. However, don't be driven by this in its totality. If you do that, you are likely to risk an overfocus on an outcome-based, performance-orientated goal. Remember the importance of process even when setting specific outcome goals.

Be patient
Take time to allow progress and focus on the process of your training. Everything will ebb and flow as you make your way through your training.

Goal setting gives you focus, process, purpose. But it doesn't actually make you *do* stuff. You have to take care of that part yourself.

That's where motivation comes in.

MOTIVATION

In the midpack, we are all runners for different reasons. We run for health, for fitness, for performance, for connection, friendships, adventure, to escape, for social reasons, to get time to ourselves, it's part of our routine, it reduces stress... Sometimes we run because of all of these things combined.

We call it mojo. What's yours and how is it?

Ask anyone in the midpack who's been injured or unable to run for a while and they will tell you how desperate they are to run. The fact that running and deciding to run is out of their hands unleashes a whole new desire to be running. The deeper aspect of this is probably linked to identity: 'I don't even feel like a runner any more'. It's when you have nothing working against you that it comes down to mojo. What's your motivation like and what shapes it?

What happens if I lose my mojo?

Losing your mojo isn't that fleeting 'I can't be arsed' feeling when the weather is bad or you've been held up at work. It's not those occasional missed runs in a training cycle, or the times you can't be bothered to go to parkrun because 9 a.m. on a Saturday isn't a great time for you. Losing your mojo is that extended period of time when you can't motivate yourself to run and you can't even see the point. For some midpack runners, mojo is sometimes lost when they get out of routine, especially following injury or illness. Going from what sometimes feels like a regimented routine to being unable to run can be difficult to get over and restart, especially if you lost fitness in that time. Equally, that mojo can vanish when runners have been overdoing it, especially overdoing the same things, in the same ways, for a prolonged period of time.

Regaining mojo: the fix!

Sometimes running mojo takes a dive. For all sorts of reasons. First, acknowledge when that happens. You've probably felt it coming. Often, you know it because you hit a performance plateau, things stop going well, start getting worse, keep getting shittier, and there's no obvious reason. Dips and troughs happen in running and when they do, mojo collapses. But it needn't. This commonly shows that your motivations, orientations and expectations are set wrong and perhaps you'd benefit from reflecting on these. Sometimes you're just tired, twitchy, irritable, stressed, frustrated, overtrained, stale and f'ed off. Let's get that mojo back and keep it under control. Don't lose the motivation to stay motivated. Help yourself get through the hump and press the reset button by waiting for the 'click'. Here are some ideas:

- Without doubt the most important thing to revitalise your mojo is patience. All too often, runners want it before its ready. You want the cake before it's baked. Wait for the mojo to click back in. It will do, but only if you wait, patiently. If you don't fancy running, then don't run. Don't force it. It's your body and brain telling you it's done for a while. Hang fire. Wait for things (energy levels, enthusiasm, recovery, focus, direction and purpose) to ignite again. When they do, you'll be ready to resume. Force it and you'll stutter and take another dive.

- Change it up. Do something different. Variety helps. If you're a runner who's hit a plateau and stalemate with your running, then there's a chance it's because you like things on repeat. Repeat gets boring. Spice it up a touch. Change your training.

- Be exciting and adventurous. Start to carve out a different approach to your running that really values how your running serves you. Reflect and realise what it gives you. When it's not there, you'll miss it. Discover something in your running that sparks your desire and passion and cultivate more of it. Do it with more purpose. Be really intentionally challenging, changing, revealing and adventurous (now we sound like marriage counsellors!).

- Use your running to serve others. Volunteer at a race. Seeing others achieving their goals can motivate you to go and get one for yourself. See volunteering as a part of you as runner. It's not a 'sacrifice' or a thankless task. It's an essential, valued and important part of contributing to a community and makes you and those around you feel better!

- Be naked. Stop worrying about pace and distance. Take your watch off for a week or two. Run when you like, as fast as you like, as far as you want.

- Explore. Run somewhere new. Choose a beautiful place and go and run there. Ignite your passion for being outside; it's there in everyone.

- Talk. Call on a friend. Be honest, tell them you're struggling. Having a buddy to meet up with makes you accountable and running together usually allows for a good switch-off from worrying about pace.

What if I feel like a failure?

Sometimes not achieving something can stop you in your tracks and make you feel like you've failed. (Even though we know, and you probably do too, that you haven't.) It sometimes happens because a goal or challenge was just too big, or your body broke down, or some other outside influence happened that changed your plans and hopes, or sometimes it's down to your perceptions of what success means and how you define it. If you set your standards unrealistically high, suffer from radical goal creep, keep moving the finish line, then are you really surprised when you're hard on yourself and are quick to call yourself a 'failure' (when you're not)?

We've heard people such as experienced ultra runner Mimi Anderson talk emotionally about failure, in her case the emotions she felt when she was unable to complete her run across the USA due to injury. On a much smaller scale, Anji has failed to finish a half marathon, despite training having gone to plan, due to her being unwell on the day and having to 'walk it in' from mile 4 (6.4km). Martin experienced what it's like to have to abandon a big challenge when he had to stop his attempt to run the entire South West Coast Path in 2016, following injuries and a few logistical problems at the start. Were any of us failures? We all believe at the start – as long as our self-talk is good – that there is a good chance we can do it. But a big challenge brings with it a level of understanding that it might not (in fact, it probably won't) go to plan. This is what makes a challenge, challenging. If we knew we could achieve it, it wouldn't be exciting or challenging. This is where your self-awareness, emotion regulation, your ability to choose a response and your skills of reflection need to come in. Looking back at what you felt challenged by, how you responded when you were challenged and how much of that was in (or not) your control are your biggest powers in framing this as a learning experience rather than a failure per se, and allowing you to grow and move on. Using and trusting in the process really helps you to reframe and redefine what success means to you, even if it's not quite what you aspired to or expected. If it is embraced, this can really help you to move through the midpack, and it's a key part of mastery.

MASTERY

Mastery is your secret weapon in the midpack. It's about growing in confidence and becoming highly motivated through mastering something – anything from dealing with something messy in your head to pacing a great track session or nailing a race confidently. We're going to refer to the act of 'mastering' something as 'mastery'. Mastery means having invested time and effort into cultivating an approach to being the runner you want to be. This could be the development of comprehensive knowledge or skill in an area, and for the midpack runner that might be mastering coping strategies to deal with any of the mind-bending things above. It's mastery of your running sessions, knowing how to execute them with purpose, knowing how to refine them, it's having the right tools to deal with negative thoughts if things don't go to plan, knowing how to regulate

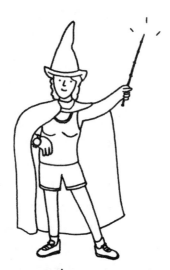

Mastery; your midpack magic wand.

your emotions and setting clear and challenging goals. It's mastery of getting your workouts 'right' and knowing how to execute a plan on race day.

Mastery takes time. But it's worth it. Mastery doesn't necessarily mean excellence and that's a really important distinction. Learning doesn't need to be, and arguably shouldn't be, about striving for perfection (we've spoken about the pitfalls of that) or about fanatical obsession (yeah, those pitfalls too). Developing a mastery mindset means that you are capable of facing the challenge, being resilient enough to stick with the challenge, being kind enough to yourself to admit vulnerabilities, being accountable enough to yourself and others, being present enough to focus on the how and the now, and being patient enough to allow the process to take care of itself.

Great mastery requires you to have a great focus and drive that comes from inside of you. Many of you may be driven, passionate people but you might experience times when that's pressed or pinched other areas of your life. We are going to look at how you deal with those in the next chapter on whole body health. Remaining driven yet patient through difficult times is key to mastery and both are found when you start to trust the process and focus on process above outcome.

We want you to stop beating yourself up if you're not the best (or even *your* best) – it's that perfection thing again. Instead of worrying about being the best or *your* best, focus on getting better. Remember, mastery requires failure to happen sometimes because when things don't work out as we hoped, planned or expected, this gives us our greatest learning experiences – so don't be scared of it. Be patient, be present and mastery will come.

JUDGEMENT

In the midpack, it can sometimes feel like we are being judged and that judgement is coming at us from a variety of angles. We might judge ourselves against others, feel judgement from friends and family (those who run, and those who don't). We sometimes feel judged by our colleagues, our coaches and even our watches and training logs with their on-screen, flashing reminders that we've done or not done something better, or worse, or the same, as the last time we did it.

In the midpack, you don't have the luxury of running being a vocation. You can't explain yourself by saying 'it's my job to run at silly o'clock, for sometimes ridiculous distances, in really shit weather'. So it's likely you'll get some raised eyebrows or comments from your non-running colleagues who might suggest that what you do is a little unhinged. Some people might not even drive in a week as far as you run on a Sunday, so in that context it might just appear bonkers that you really, truly, are doing it for fun and because you love it.

You might have family members who cast judgement on what you're doing, and really, you can't blame them. Training for something big that completely immerses you can have the effect of turning you into a bore. We think this is the reason runners gravitate together. They are the people most likely to understand all the early starts, missed social events, time spent, money spent. It might be that we'd even run less frequently if we were always surrounded by non-runners.

But judgement from others might be nothing compared to the way you judge yourself – it's that perfectionist runner thing again! Unchecked, we can become our worst critics and this can get out of hand. We pass judgement, often based on a number on a clock or through those dreaded words on Strava 'This run trending slower', but we also make these judgements based on a whole bunch of 'what ifs'. Judgement is uncomfortable because it can make you feel embarrassed, humiliated and rejected.

Avoiding judgement either from ourselves – comparing ourselves to when we were younger, fitter, faster – or from others, who might discuss our race times or roll their eyes at us behind our backs, can mean we sometimes wrap ourselves up in smaller, less scary targets. This can mean you surround yourself with doubt and fear and spend too long within your comfort zone. We want you to address how you respond to judgment so that you're not tempted to stay there.

Control how you respond: the fix

Being happy, present, content and non-judgemental of yourself (and of others) is a really important part of being a midpack runner. But it's tricky; being judgemental and making unhelpful comparisons with yourself and with others can hurt and so often is wrapped up in much deeper emotional issues than we are capable of exploring in this running book. When you frame your running results, identity and friendships in a big bunch of performance-orientated outcomes, and throw in some perfectionist tendencies, sprinkle on some insecurities and anxieties and drop on a hefty lump of self-criticism, it's not surprising running can become harmful over helpful. Running gives you so much, but if you're easily judgemental of yourself or others, don't let judgement fuel anger or anxiety. Instead, it's time to get more compassionate and be more open (let's hug). Here are some pointers:

- See things from others' point of view – if you're feeling judged by others in your running, try to see it from their point of view and consider how you can fix things to help you both understand. Listen, seek to understand.

- Other people's opinions might be none of your business – if you feel you're being judged harshly, for example on your race performances, consider that their opinion won't make any difference to you unless you let it. You choose your response. Don't let any negative judgement impact on what you do next.

- Be kinder to yourself – notice when you are feeling judged, or when you are tempted to judge others. See how it makes you feel. Be more compassionate, softer and patient with yourself.

- Learn to accept compliments – it's not always easy to accept compliments about your running. When someone says to you 'Hey, well done today, you looked strong', your judgmental self may instinctively reach for the perfectionist, self-critical response that you 'should have run faster, could have shaved off those extra seconds, or not walked up that hill'. Put that on hold and graciously accept the compliment with a 'thank you'.

When judgement and comparison hurts

It would be naive of us to not acknowledge the harmful significance and danger of judgement and comparison when desires to achieve a time, body image, size or shape become uncontrollably unhealthy. We know this happens, we know we want to mention it, we know it's relevant and impacts many people, some of whom you'll never know. We also know we can't do the issues full justice within the confines and context of this book. However, if you're reading this and things resonate, we encourage you to talk and seek support.

Next time you casually flick through your Instagram feed and notice it's full of shiny, athletic, fast-looking people, hold the scroll and check your inner personal comparison filters.

Body dysmorphic disorder

Body dysmorphic disorder (BDD) is closely linked to self-esteem, perfectionism and confidence. BDD is more than just that fleeting 'I'm feeling a little fat' thing that might come and go for some of you if you have a few less active weeks or feel a little bloated. BDD is not an eating disorder, but some people with BDD might suffer from some disordered eating. We are going to talk a little more about food and RED-S (relative energy deficiency in sport) in Chapter 5 and why for some people in the midpack eating can get a little messy and unhealthy.

BDD is much more likely to be ongoing rather than a passing feeling that comes and goes, and instead presents as a huge anxiety about appearance, a fixation on perceived flaws that probably only you can see. While BDD might for some people be an obsession with having a nose that they see as imperfect or ears that are a bit too big, in running it can be worrying when it links to your body, your weight, seeing yourself as 'fat', 'too thin', 'too big to run', 'not muscular enough to run' or something else that drives you to want to develop unhealthy eating or exercise routines as you strive for perceived perfection. People with BDD are often highly critical of themselves and will often isolate themselves from others because they feel ashamed. We've seen runners with this disorder who, among other things, become obsessed with their race photos, develop unhealthy routines with food, get highly anxious about wearing (or not wearing) a particular type of kit, right along to someone who avoided doing a particular exercise in the gym because they felt people would be looking at them.

Dr Simon Marshall describes body dysmorphic disorder (BDD) as overwhelming feelings of negative thoughts, usually related to perceived flaws in physical appearance that don't seem to really relate to how you look to other people. It's important to recognise that BDD is an anxiety disorder that, according to Simon, is often: 'accompanied by a psychiatric shit storm of other conditions', such as depression, a dependency on exercise, obsessive compulsive disorder and eating disorders. However, Simon says BDD is 'pretty rare among runners because there is almost always something else going on, for example, secondary exercise dependence and that would not be classified as BDD.'

The charity MIND (www.mind.org.uk) has a list of suggestions for how to look for BDD in yourself and others and explains that many will avoid getting help in case they are seen as being vain. MIND lists symptoms of BDD, such as an obsession with a perceived flaw or flaws in physical appearance, including being too big or too small, or having an area that you might see as being out of proportion. It's really important to address this if you feel it's an issue for you that might be affecting how you're training or eating, or if you think someone close to you has it. Don't go in all guns blazing; ask questions of yourself and others that are kind and have good intentions. If you're concerned about someone else, start by saying you're a little worried about them, and mention some of the behaviours you've noticed. Make sure they know this is coming from a good place and that they can trust you. You can't force someone to get help, but you can show support and share concerns that might allow them to open up and start the steps towards becoming a happier and healthier human being.

SOCIAL MEDIA PRESSURES

The only way you won't feel any of the pressure of social media is to not be on social media! Anji has spent half of the time she's been a runner working in social media and we have both seen the greatness of it, as well as witnessing sometimes first-hand how it can be destructive. Social media gives everyone a voice and a platform on which to share an opinion; it's a great tool for building community, sharing experiences, creating bonds, telling stories, keeping up to date, learning and networking. However, without accountability, preservation, boundaries and a thick skin, sometimes it can be harmful to your running head.

Start by considering how much you really use social media. How many times do you actively use it every day? And what are you really using social media for? Think about it.

How social media are you?

- I track what I am doing.
- I track what I am doing, and I look at what other people are doing.
- I track what I am doing, I look at what other people are doing, I interact with what other people are doing.
- I track what I am doing, I look at what other people are doing, I interact with what other people are doing, I compare what I do with what other people are doing.
- I track what I am doing, I look at what other people are doing, I interact with what other people are doing, I compare what I do with what other people are doing, I seek approval from others for what I have been doing.
- I track what I am doing, I look at what other people are doing, I interact with what other people are doing, I compare what I do with what other people are doing, I seek approval from others for what I have been doing. I feel rewarded, encouraged, positive about myself, affirmed and happy. I feel frustrated, disappointed, anxious, angry, upset with myself.

The anti-social media – the problem

Ask yourself, how much of what you are digesting (and sharing) online is not just good, but really great? We wonder if Pheidippides would have completed the first ever marathon if he'd had one eye on his splits, worrying how it would look on Strava when he was, actually, going to die. It's a good exercise to take stock of what you are using, how often you use it and the positive effect, if any, it's having on your running and you, the midpack runner.

Social media pressures can distract many of us – elites included. Former GB international 1500m athlete Colin McCourt has seen both sides of social media, first using it as a massive motivator to track his journey back to fitness for a 5km (3.1-mile) challenge to run under 16 minutes for 5k in 2017. Colin regularly shared videos, training sessions and results as he trained hard and interacted with a supportive community that willed him on. If we open ourselves up in this way on social media it can be a brilliant motivator as you have a community there at hand if you want to build one, who will cheer you on from wherever they are in the world. The flip side of this is that sometimes it can have the opposite effect. It is at worst a comparison tool you have in your hand at any time of day to show you what others are doing when you are not (or can't!). Colin told us that social media was also destructive for him as he became wrapped up in competition and ultimately controlled by the desire for likes, kudos, any digital thumbs-up he could get his hands on. The fix for Colin was to get back to his own driven mindset, which had made him a champion in the first place, and focus on himself, saying: 'The only way to be is to be yourself. What others do is amazing but it doesn't define your training, or even you.'

If it's dragging you down, it's good to look at social media as a highlights reel. For many, their social media feed is often a way of showing the times when they did something great, or looked great, ran a time they were proud of. Dr Simon Marshall says it's natural to want to share your highlights: 'For most of us, your brain is wired to curate a history of yourself or a presentation of yourself that's going to appeal and make you the most attractive, fast, shaggable … all the things that evolutionists told us are good characteristics. We do it all the time.' Nobody is ever going to put the full picture out there – they wouldn't have time to, anyway. Accept that comparing your bad days to someone else's best days isn't going to help you to feel better.

The anti-social media – the fix

There's one really straightforward fix to your social media dilemmas. Come off social media. Bin it. Leave all your social platforms permanently. That might be a little harsh for some, and we admit that social media platforms and their relative functionality can enhance and enrich runners' experiences, but it's a minefield that you need to carefully and competently navigate your way through. If you do decide to stay on social media, you should try to do the following:

Cultivate progress, nourish achievement, bring joy

Learn to filter
Effective filtering could mean cultivating your social feeds to be helpful and constructive (cull negative or unhelpful people or feeds, harshly where necessary) but also applying your own internal nonsense filter. If you don't like it, you don't have to engage with it. Don't allow yourself to get sucked in. Use your social media experience to add and improve your online and offline running experience.

Digital detox
Martin likes to set defined periods during which he steps away from social media either entirely, or a platform at a time. For Anji, having a locked and private Strava account is the game changer. Not looking at anyone else's training and not worrying about outside judgement makes it much more healthy for her to crack on.

Stop comparing yourself to others
You know by now that everyone in the midpack is completely different. That's what's great about it. You're never going to be the same as the next person based on an app you're both using.

Think of it as a highlights reel
Remind yourself that others are having bad days too, they're just not talking about it online.

Throughout this book, we consistently reinforce the importance of engaging with and learning to love the process of running. It's this understanding that will help you gain more from the running that you do currently, make the most of your running in the future and establish a meaningful and sustainable life-enhancing relationship with the world of running and the people you share it with. Ryan Hall, 2.04 marathoner, summed this up beautifully in a 'Marathon Talk' interview (Episode 481, 27.3.19):

> 'I think it's a culture of learning to enjoy the process, enjoy the journey, and it's something that has to be cultivated every single day. You've got to water it, give it sunshine, or else it's not going to grow. It's a mindset. It's not a one-time shift, it's an over and over again. In an ideal world, it's about surrounding yourself with a community that holds the same values, knows that it's about process. It's not about comparing yourself to other people, comparing yourself to your former self, your previous self. It's about loving the process.'

The simplicity of the act of doing the 'how' of your running, the love for the 'what' you do and the joy of participating in it, is what will help you progress *on your terms* in the midpack. For some, that will at times mean extra effort, more time, greater personal investment, significant emotional attachment and a purposeful physical pressure. By contrast, at times, or for others, the emphasis will be different, less outcome focussed, more emergent, more relational, richer yet just as rewarding.

In this chapter, we've dug into giving yourself permission and specifically how, if you let it, running can mess with your head, a little, or a lot. Yet we hope we've shown you that it's possible to cultivate running progress through raising your understanding of how your mind works to boost or sabotage your running, to create the strongest mental climates for your running to thrive, and to help you know how to nourish your running achievements by applying yourself diligently, building and maintaining effective confidence, regulating your emotions with regard to generating anxiety, pressure or being judgemental, and making difficult comparisons. When you focus on the small how-to steps of process over a big must-do performance-oriented outcome then the pathway to your personally defined success, and a desirable outcome, is smoother, easier to manage, simpler to cope with, stronger and more likely to produce a happier experience of running and moving in the midpack that will bring joy to your running.

THREE

WHOLE BODY HEALTH

LOVE YOUR BODY

Being a better midpack runner is about so much more than just running. If you think you can hammer your running self and move up through the midpack (if that's what you want to achieve) then you'd better think again. We value your health as a whole human being over your 'running performance' stats and status. We want you to love running, love your body, value your participation, be able to run how you want to run – today, tomorrow and for many years into the future.

In this chapter, we are going to guide you gently away from running and towards the bigger picture of your overall health and wellness. We have written much more about your mental health in Chapter 2 and nutrition in Chapter 5, so here we're going to take you through preventing and dealing with injury, becoming a generally more robust runner, why rest is a vital part of your training, how to accept the pressures of everyday life, and a little bit of snuggly, tree-hugging self-care. We are going to frame that self-care in some good, purposeful rest and recovery, and we are going to show you why it's great to work on your weaknesses with some strength and conditioning exercises in your plan.

It's all part of the process.

Your whole body health should always come back to the pillars of performance that make you able to train at all. To keep the plates spinning and for you to be able to actually 'do' running, you first have to look at those pillars properly. On the foundations of your family, general life, health and work, you're (trying to) build everything else on top of recovery, rest, nutrition and your mental health and emotional state. You wouldn't be human if there wasn't something that felt a bit wobbly.

We want you to view your running in a much bigger frame, and see that while it isn't the be-all and end-all, it can positively shape a large part of your identity, and there are so many things you can do that will make you a better, happier member of the midpack.

How would you define your current well-being? For me (Martin), certainly over the years this is something that has changed. As a young person, I think my well-being wasn't something I particularly paid much attention to unless I was unwell. In my 20s and 30s, my personal well-being was much more aligned with improving athletic performance. Was I well enough to push physical boundaries, to ask more of an exercising body, to go faster, harder, longer? Looking back, and with a degree of hindsight, I'd argue that much of the life of an elite athlete is contrary to overall holistic well-being.

Currently, my well-being means so much more to me. It's about my whole body: physical, mental and emotional health, the ability to be *more than* functional every day, to flourish in the world, to be able to run and play with my kids, to have an absence of ill health, to feel fulfilled, to have a sense of purpose, to feel valued and secure, to live in contentment, to live a life of quality for longer. What wellness and well-being means is highly personal, situational and contextual, but most people can agree that good well-being is about finding a health balance that allows you to define 'what matters most' to you. If you're reading this, then like me, I imagine that your physical and mental wellness are important parts of your overall framework of well-being.

As a regular midpack runner, my overall well-being is shaped by physical activity through running. If you could imagine your well-being as a house, physical and mental health are the roof. Having a roof over your head is the most important part of well-being, but good roofs are supported by walls (or in this case, pillars). Yet wellness in these contexts is also supported by the ability to manage important pillars of physical and mental well-being. To make sure that the core supports for my roof are strong, I need to be continually supportive of my overall well-being; I must pay close attention to the stability and strength of the pillars that support it; for example, rest, recovery, sleep, nutrition, whole body conditioning, reduced stress, lifestyle.

These important pillars don't exist in isolation. They are all related and interact. The relationship between them isn't simple, but the integration of each does shape wellness and how we feel. From personal experience, I know that it's hard to integrate them seamlessly and effectively when 'life' throws up uncertainties, pressure points and problems.

For me (Anji), my current well-being seems to shift regularly and often as a result of stress. I have always been a midpack runner and approaching my 40s, I now have a handle on managing my health much better than when I started running in my late 20s. All I wanted to do then was run, run faster and be lighter than I was in order to do so. I was driven to be the best runner I could be and the slimmest I could manage, often with dangerously unhealthy rituals at play, while at the same time holding down a very stressful job I didn't enjoy that required me to work long hours. My way of dealing with stress, rather than any sort of self-care, was just to keep training more.

Progressing into my 30s, changing jobs, changing everything, dealing with long-term injury and illness, and beginning to address my body image issues changed my well-being entirely. I sleep better, I eat better, my running is better because I look after it better, especially when it comes to training in a more purposeful, structured and strength-focused way. I still don't have all the answers, but I am kinder to myself than the old me was.

Like Martin, I am far better now at seeing myself as 'whole' and keeping the pillars as strong as possible, especially when it comes to rest, sleep and how I react to stress.

It's really important for overall well-being to develop self-awareness of your instability triggers. When one pillar starts to shake, what are the warning signs? How can you tell when that pillar is becoming unstable, what action can you take to settle the wobble and regain composure, integration and pillar stability? For example, a work or a relationship pressure point can cause disruption across several pillars: you lose sleep, you get more stressed, your nutrition takes a dive. This disruption isn't sustainable; cracks in the pillars are manageable up to a point, with careful support, but longer-term weakness, gaping holes and collapse in one or more pillars can lead to significant negative impact on overall well-being.

Running can be a valuable glue that connects and supports your pillars. Learning to let running and exercise be a strength and a support rather than a means of weakening pillars is really important.

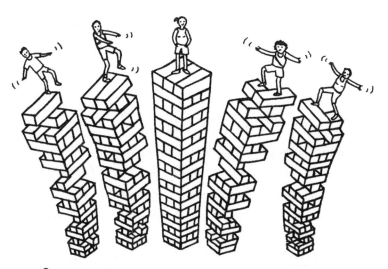

Stable pillars = strong foundations.

Let's look at some core pillars and how to keep them strong and stable. We are going to get into the key areas of rest and recovery, with some tips to help you to sleep better, as well as exploring why it's so important. We are going to talk about getting strong with some examples of exercises and easy ways of dropping strength into your regular routine. We are going to look at stretching, running technique, female health and cycles, and what we call 'stress buttons'. We are going to get you to think about how you react to stress and injury and walk you through how to deal with those pressures in a way that is positive and reflective.

REST AND RECOVERY – WHO IS REALLY GETTING IT?

Who in the midpack is really, honestly, getting loads of great sleep? We have our busy lives, our stresses, our shift patterns, our kids, and somewhere beyond those things we have our running. It might look like it to our family and friends sometimes, but running doesn't always come first, and nor should it. We aren't going to harp on at you about how important sleep is. You know you should be getting it, and you probably know that it's one of your real secret weapons in the midpack. You can get yourself the best trainers, spend a whole heap of cash on the best recovery drinks on the market and treat yourself to a sports massage once a week, but they're unlikely to give you the same benefits as some regular decent sleep.

Snooze your way through the midpack

Moving through the midpack is built on maintaining strong pillars of wellness, and without doubt sleep is one the pillar bad boys. Training (oh, and life, right!) places tough physical demands on the body. In fact, regular training actually breaks down the body and it is during recovery and rest periods that adaptation and so-called 'training effect' takes place. Yes, that's right, runners get fitter, stronger and faster as a result of training that includes, rather than overlooks, proper recovery. Recovery includes nutrition and rest but it's during sleep and in particular 'deep sleep' that the greatest physiological repair and regeneration takes place and restoration and revitalisation peaks. Growth hormones are released during this phase, and the body's metabolism is functioning at a rate that enables healing, growth and repair to occur most effectively. Without this period of restorative sleep, the body is unable to restore itself optimally and effectively and can leave you feeling tired and fatigued for your next run.

Getting regular deep sleep isn't as easy as it sounds and many of us suffer with broken and irregular sleeping patterns due to work, lifestyle and family commitments. Poor-quality sleep really isn't great for optimum recovery from regular running. In fact, as we age, the amount of time we are able to spend enjoying the benefits of 'high-quality deep sleep' actually deteriorates. While 10-year olds spend 25 per cent of their sleep in deep sleep, by the time we reach 40 this figure has dropped to 10 per cent for men and 12 per cent for women. So, as we get older, it becomes increasingly more important to bag the early nights after a hard day's running. It makes sense for runners to spend as much time as possible in deep restorative sleep in order to get the most of their running training and be up, ready and focused for everyday training. Without doubt, high-quality sleep helps runners perform better, have higher energy levels, recover stronger and run faster.

Sleep strong, run strong – our kip tips

1. Be comfortable – not all of us can sleep on a stick and so good bedding, a comfortable bed and an optimum sleep environment are all important to ensure a great night's sleep.

2. Grab an extra hour – go to bed an extra hour early at least two days of the week. Make a conscious effort to get to bed earlier or stay in bed later. The additional time spent recovering will reap dividends when the training picks up.

3. Screens off – turn off TVs, laptops, monitors and screens at least 60 minutes before your head hits the pillow. Give your eyes time to refocus and tune out before getting into bed.

4. Don't make a meal of it – try not to have your biggest meal of the day late at night and then hop straight into the sack. Leave at least 90 minutes–2 hours after eating before going to bed.

5. Unwind – after a hard training session your body is probably 'up' and even though you feel tired, your mind may be awake. Before getting into bed, give your body and mind a good few hours to relax and unwind and for that adrenaline to dissipate.

The importance of rest

Rest *is* training. Oh yes, you read that right. A healthy body needs rest during sleep *and* during the day. Rest is something we want you to look at differently. Please start regarding it as something you should be doing, you give yourself permission to do, you don't feel guilty or anxious about, and regularly, purposefully and carefully plan it into your self-care routine.

A rest day should be just that. They are, believe it or not, for resting. They're not days-off-running days, otherwise that's what they'd be called. Rest days allow your body to repair properly, and that's the key reason they are important for your training. Don't get rest confused with cross-training, hill climbing, bike riding, weight lifting and even going for that 'leisurely swim'. All of these are great if they are your thing, but let's be clear, they are not resting. Rest shouldn't be mistaken for a reduction in activity or a time to do something else (and that includes that massive DIY task that's been hanging around).

When to plan high quality 'rich rest' hinges on the integration of your running into your lifestyle. A good running plan and routine will see you plan rest in both when it is required and also when it is not required. You shouldn't wait until you have to take enforced rest. Enforced rest happens when you haven't listened to your body, when your wellness pillars have weakened, when you've overcooked and overcommitted. Enforced rest means you've broken when you didn't want to. Careful, tactical rest is planned, purposeful, productive, fruitful, enjoyable, and happens as a part of your life. When you can effortlessly plan rest into your schedule it demonstrates that you are in control of your running rather than your running being in control of you. Rich rest leaves you feeling refreshed, revitalised, focused, energised, ready for your next run, or certainly ready to tackle the next day ahead of you.

We don't all rest the same. Some people are better default 'resters' than others. They just take to it better, respond better and enjoy it more. Others struggle to shoe horn rest into their schedules. Importantly, it's up to you to understand where and how rest fits (could fit, or should fit) into your life and to prioritise real rest as a vital part of the maintenance and stability of your pillars of well-being.

One of the best pieces of advice we have been given came from Professor Andy Lane, who said runners should try to even *think* differently on rest days. Use them to do anything and everything that takes you away from your identity as a runner, and brings you back to just being you. Andy suggests proactive planning – putting effort into trying to do something interesting means you might not even have time to think about running.

This is really important. Rest is much more than physical state. It's also about a mental and emotional break and recovery, calm away from the business of your life, space from pressures, change, motivational maintenance, focus switching, and comfort in allowing yourself a time-out.

Rest days aren't there for worrying about a race, logistically planning your next event or reflecting on your training last week. They should be a total switch-off and, in time, when you are really used to them, they should become glorious and much-anticipated days in your plan. There should be no more 'winging it' with rest days than there is for 'training days', and as with anything else in your plan, they should be regular, purposeful, planned and specific: specifically doing nothing related to running.

The mindset of a great rester isn't anything too virtuous, it's more a simple confidence that comes from knowing this chance to recover properly will lead to a greater gain in training – and isn't that what we all want? Good resters aren't sitting around thinking how great it is to sit on their arse (although, it kind of is), they are in fact taking the rest in the same way they take in a great session or a long run. It just matters.

When and how many rest days you should have each week is something you need to practise and get right, and this will vary massively between runners in the midpack depending on the job you do, what you are training for and other things, such as your lifestyle and overall health. As a general rule, you should start with at least one complete rest day per week. As with most things, your life will dictate this and it's certainly worth considering if you are still feeling exhausted and broken that you need to look at when, how and how often you are 'doing' rest.

Note: if resting comes a little too naturally to you, it's just as important to plan rest days in so you're not tempted to just take one every day at the expense of actually running…

GET STRONG – MAKING YOURSELF BULLET-PROOF WITHOUT BEING ARNIE

Strength and conditioning (S&C) isn't something that's always been recognised for the midpack runner, but it's another element of running – like some of the stuff we are going to talk about Chapter 4 – that might just make a difference. Doing the same things all of the time gets the same results all of the time. Some of you may say that you just don't have the time for S&C, some might fear 'bulking up' as a product of lifting weights, while for others it's simply a matter of lack of desire to go to a gym when running otherwise gives us complete freedom. So let's be clear: getting stronger as a runner isn't going to make you bulky, or slow you down. Good strength and conditioning for you is purposeful, relevant, functional and focused and should mean you become slightly more bullet-proof, a better and stronger runner who is less likely to become injured, or less likely to have repeated injuries. You should be able to train for longer periods without the interruption of breaking down, allowing you to make the gains you want towards your goal race, time or event.

Short version: it's worth doing.

Running and doing nothing else can get you specifically 'run strong', but complementing your running with functional S&C can help you hit that PB. Running specialist physiotherapist Paul Hobrough, author of *The Runner's Expert Guide to Stretching* (Bloomsbury), sees runners with a massive range of experience, including many from the midpack, often when they are at the stage of breaking down physically. 'Running is arguably only strengthening you in a very specific, repeated muscle pattern, so the stimulus for strength growth and injury resilience is lost once you reach a programme you are used to. Of course, you can change your runs about a little, which will have some effect, but essentially, you are, at a certain point in your running journey, just maintaining your standard, so you cannot expect to achieve a new PB,' says Paul. We see this a lot in the midpack, and often it comes from just getting a little too comfortable, set in routine, doing the same things all of the time because we like it that way. Commonly, runners seek pure consistency without a lot of change in the pursuit of progress and some can even fear adding or changing that routine too much. But it's worth it!

'The route to a new PB is a new training load and the path to being bullet-proof against injury is found through strengthening not only the prime movers but the accessory muscles of the body,' states Paul.

It's the route to a PB. Have we got your attention now?

Moving in the midpack and getting 'better' at your running, whether that's in the progress you make or in your general happiness as a runner, requires something of a commitment to some good functional strength work. Again, this is about the process and what you learn along the way, putting your faith into doing something new or differently and trusting that it will lead you to better results. Anji was one of those midpack runners who was a little scared of breaking routine by adding strength work into her training, but after embracing it in the last three years, she has found that she has broken down much less regularly and, most importantly, has been able to train through cycles for longer, without the disruption of niggles. Consider the potential of how great it can be if it's done in a measured and careful way before haphazardly starting a strength regime that will only give you random guns that probably only you will be impressed by anyway.

BUILD A MORE ROBUST BODY WITH SIMPLE STUFF

While it's true that you might need a gym or some equipment at home in order to progress strength work, there are quite a few exercises you can add to your routine that involve just you and your body weight. The great thing about starting with the basics is that they don't take too long and can be done at home.

The basics

These are the bread-and-butter elements of strength work. They are minimal in terms of time and equipment required, but maximal in what they can give you back in return if done regularly and progressively. They are:

- Calf raises
- Squats
- Dead lifts
- Pull-ups
- Planks
- Sit-ups
- Press-ups

The next level

These exercises move you up a notch. They are often added to create a longer routine of strength or to progress to something a little more difficult once you've mastered the basics:

- Resistance bands – adding stretchy bits of rubber with increasing grades of intensity to your arms/legs to create resistance when performing an exercise.

- Drills – repeated exercises that focus on skills such as balance and agility. Sometimes done with hurdles, cones or a flat 'ladder'.

WTF

This is the stuff that might seem a little weird at first glance. You might feel awkward doing these, but the pay-off is definitely worth it. They build power, agility and poise when done regularly:

- Calisthenics – repeated, rhythmic movement exercises using only body weight.
- Plyometrics – exercises that often incorporate jumping or 'bounding' to use large muscles at maximum impact, such as jumping sideways or up on to a high box.

The best thing is to resist the urge to just do exercises from one these groups, and instead put together something with a strength coach that allows you to do a bit of all of them. We hear of fabled midpack runners who never get injured (?!) but the truth is there's nobody in the midpack who should be neglecting strength work completely.

Like rest days, 'doing' strength should be planned, purposeful and specific, and for it to really make a difference, it should be progressive, too. That might mean adding physical weights, such as barbells, dumb-bells and Olympic bars, to exercises you previously only used body weight for, increasing the weight you have been using on a bar, or jumping up on to a higher box if you are doing plyometrics.

Make sure your strength sessions – whatever they look like to you – fit in where you have the best chance of forming a habit to actually do them, and not on a rest day! It shouldn't end up being something else you don't do and just feel guilty about; you possibly have enough stuff to feel inferior about without this. This should go without saying, but strength sessions shouldn't come the day before your big speed workout, long run or race. As with resting, strength fits best if the timing is right to allow your body to make the training gains and correctly recover from them. We recommend sandwiching some strength between your faster days, your easy runs, and a couple of days before you plan to rest.

Top strength exercises to make you bullet-proof

Build a strong core and stronger legs and the results will follow. These are the exercises to focus on:

- Heel raises
- Squats
- Dead lifts
- Split squats
- Crab walks
- Single-leg squats
- Single-leg dead lifts
- Pull-ups
- Press-ups
- Clams
- Glute bridges
- Chest presses
- Russian twists
- Step-ups
- Box jumps
- Aleknas
- Dead bugs

Note: Mix and match, and never do them all on one day! As a starting point, we suggest choosing six of these exercises and doing them as a circuit at least once a week. A good 20–30-minute circuit would be 8–12 repetitions (reps) of each one, up to three times with plenty of rest in between. You'll find some of them harder than others and that's OK. Just keep track of what starts to feel easier and add progressions to the exercises using weights or bands.

If you've never done any strength work before, it's really important to frame it positively as an important and worthwhile addition to your running. It might feel odd at first, and if you are changing anything you might ache a bit in a different way than you are used to, but bank this as part of a process that will make you a better, more robust runner.

AND STRETCH...

Mention stretching in a group of midpack runners and you'll get some mixed reactions. We've met some dedicated stretchers in the midpack, many of whom embrace yoga or specific stretching sessions and tell us it's the best addition they made to their running. We've also met runners with hamstrings so inflexible we worry they might just snap like a stick if they bend at the waist to tie a shoelace. The main things we are asked about stretching are always when it should be done (pre/post run or both), how long each stretch should take, what are the 'main' stretches they should do, and also if there's really any benefit to it. Paul Hobrough reported that he very rarely meets runners who stretch enough, saying: 'I'm not sure if they know what they're doing, or why they should be doing it.' He went on to explain that stretching should be seen as stretching out tight spokes on a bike, being specific, instead of globally looking to stretch everything and just doing none of it. Paul also explained that it isn't just a midpack thing, either – it's a runner thing.

So be honest. Are you stretching enough? Unless you're diligently stretching after every run, or doing yoga regularly, it's unlikely. Like some strength work, some runners might become dedicated to stretching if it helps them to recover from injury, but as soon as they are running again the good habits go out of the window. If you don't know where to start, run a stretching inventory by working through some of the key stretches, which we are coming to next, taking each side at a time, and listing where the tight spots are. Those are the areas that need the work.

We are big fans of drills that enable mobility and dynamic stretching during a warm-up (e.g. high knees, butt flicks, sideways stepping) as well as targeted stretches after your runs to tackle those weaker/problem areas that you've highlighted as in need of attention and/or simply noticed after your runs. For example, if you've got a calf that always protests the day after your long run, spend some extra time mobilising and stretching the area around the calf when you stop running. Paul Hobrough says: 'You're not going to get the best from yourself biomechanically without a prior warm-up,' and added that static stretches at the end of a run were really valuable in preventing injury (but don't do static stretches as part of your warm-up).

Strong stretch routine

After every run, it's really useful in terms of recovery and injury prevention if you spend around 10 minutes stretching. Paul Hobrough recommends building a core, simple, key stretch routine for the gastrocnemius and soleus (lower leg and calf), quad, hamstring, glute, adductors (upper leg and buttocks) and the tensor fascia latae (TFL) – this isn't a posh coffee, it's a small pelvic stability muscle located in the front of your hip. Stretching the TFL can really help to ward off injuries to areas such as the iliotibial (IT) band friction which commonly occur when the TFL becomes a little too tight.

The length of stretching time is important, too. It takes up to 6 seconds for your central nervous system to stop 'fighting' the stretch, and the ideal time per stretch is 40–60 seconds each side. Relax! It'll do you good.

RUNNING TECHNIQUE MATTERS, BUT DON'T GET HUNG UP ON IT

Good form, progressive technique work and even thinking about your poise will help you, without you needing to be a prick about it. We are both advocates of technical work – Anji is a big fan of technical drills while Martin has recently embraced calisthenics. We have both found that spending time on technique has led to improvements in our own running as well as obvious ironing-out of technique issues with the runners we coach.

Has anyone ever said to you, with the best intentions of course: 'what *is* that funny thing you do with your arms when you run? If you stopped doing it, you might run faster?' Although we might all think we glide effortlessly along when we run, the reality is that we probably don't share the same technical grace, perfect posture and fundamental good form as the world's elite. We might not even notice it until we see race photos or video. Elite runners make it all look so easy as they dance around the tracks, trails and roads. Relaxed, feet barely touching the ground, head and hips high, bodies flowing, balanced and poised. We might imagine we look like that when we run, but a cheeky glance in our reflection in a shop window as we shuffle by quickly tells us otherwise. You know what (here's the really good bit…!) – that's OK! Who gives a crap what we look like when we run? Running isn't supposed to be a form contest! It's not about what we look like when we do it, it's about how we feel and the physical, mental and social benefits.

That said, and while we don't want you to get too hung up on this, there are some instances where looking into form and technique might help. We are going to take you through how to spot if your technique is holding you back and how you can successfully tweak your form to be a better, more consistent or faster runner.

Make yourself more consistent

Getting injured is one of the biggest causes of inconsistent training and frustrated runners. Whether it's an annoying recurring niggle or a sudden unwanted acute injury, poor running form can be the culprit and more often than not making subtle changes to your running technique can be the best strategy for rehabilitation and getting back running again. The problem here lies in accurately identifying the biomechanical area of weakness, diagnosing how and why this is contributing to injury, and setting an appropriate programme of rehabilitation, conditioning and technical improvement exercises that will help address and rectify the issue. Again, ask an expert about this. Use great physios and podiatrists with good knowledge of runners (and running) to assess your imbalances and give you the best advice for how to deal with it. Shane Benzie from Running Reborn has written extensively about this in his book *The Lost Art of Running*.

Get faster, run further

Here's when better technique really starts to matter. If it's performance improvement you seek, then technique could hold the key to chopping valuable minutes and seconds off your times. Think about this in swimming terms. We've all been there. In the local leisure centre, as an injured runner, trying to maintain our fitness by trawling up and down the pool fighting the water with every stroke and thrashing as we come up for air. Working really hard but going nowhere. Then a 12-year old kid gets in and cruises past with fishlike ease. A swimmer will spend hours and hours on technical drills, learning and relearning the finer stroke elements to master different areas of their personal stroke and make them a cleaner and more efficient swimmer through the water. Swimmers learn to feel the water and to use it to their benefit. A smooth, powerful, relaxed and effective swimming technique brings both efficiency and grace to a swimmer's style and performance. We tend to not focus on that as runners. We just run.

The reality is that effective running technique actually is really important to better (and that could mean faster or further) running. For longer-distance runners, it's especially important for relaxation (both mental and physical), for efficiency and for running economy. A strong, balanced, fluid running technique creates a smooth, economical and comfortable running style. Master effective running technique and you'll not only be able to run faster but also be at less risk of injury.

How to know when to change it?

How do you know if your technique needs to change? Two things are important. First, when your style or technical quirk is energy costly and hence inefficient, this costs you time. Second, when your style causes biomechanical weakness or limitations, these can and do result in injury – this costs you training time, adaption and consistency, and is really frustrating (and potentially painful)!

We want you to recognise that there is no single correct, right or perfect way to run. No single size fits all runners, and recommendations for one runner will differ for another. Some styles and techniques are better suited to different distances or disciplines within running. For example, a high knee lift, powerful forward hip drive and fast pawing of the foot on the ground is more suited to sprinting than ultra running. If your running style doesn't cause you specific problems, isn't hugely energy inefficient and you don't get injured, then why bother breaking it down and building it back up? If you're happy with your running, are still improving, not getting injured and it's functional, specific and strong to your chosen running events then don't try to alter things. At the same time, there are a few tell-tale signs that your running technique could benefit from some help and some minor refinements could really help you be more efficient and injury-free.

Four signs that your running technique needs some help

1. You keep getting injured or have muscle soreness. There are many different reasons for getting injured but a recurring injury or niggle that simply won't go away could be down to poor running biomechanics.

2. You fatigue quickly and shuffle a lot. Do your hips drop, does your stride shorten and is your knee lift non-existent? If so, poor technique could be to blame.

3. You make a lot of noise. If as you run your feet slap loudly on the ground then this is a sure sign there is something going on further back in the run technique chain.

4. You just do that funny arm, leg, foot or head thing. You know what I'm talking about. Your arm flaps about at your side, or perhaps your knees knock together, your head bobs about, or one of your feet turns out.

LET'S NOT WAIT TO COCK IT UP

Doing rehab and strength exercises shouldn't just be a by-product of getting injured. Runners in the midpack are often guilty of waiting for the shit to hit the fan before they even consider jumping into doing strength exercises (it isn't always 'work'). That's totally understandable because in the great plate-spinning existence we live in between work, life and running, there isn't a great deal of other time. But you know the drill – prevention really is better than break, panic, google, pay a load of money to a physio, then eventually cure. 'Doing' strength work allows you to keep on top of things, making injury less likely to ever happen, or certainly happen less frequently. We call the work that goes into preventing injury 'prehab' and the work you do to get over it 'rehab'. We don't expect you to do injury rehab exercises forever, either. Anji's sports therapist once said that following multiple injuries in the past, if she did all the exercises she had ever been set there wouldn't be any time left to even go to work.

Luckily for us in the midpack, we have been running long enough to know what our weak spots are, what will be most likely to cause us to break down and, therefore, what we should be focusing on to become stronger. Think about your most recent build-up to a race and pinpoint the niggles or breakdowns you had. Training diaries are useful for this as they will also tell you when they occurred. We'll get into this in Chapter 4, too – reflection is so important. Note your hot spots, make lists if you need to, and jot down what your sweet spots are, too. You will soon see what needs to be your priority. Make this regular reflection part of the process and the routine so that it becomes habit.

It might look something like this:

February: Calf tightness (left leg) in high-rep fast session. Some hamstring tightness after long easy run (left leg).

March: Calf feeling much better, some Achilles discomfort (right leg) after parkrun.

April: Lower back pain in long runs, left side radiating into hip.

You're likely to see a pattern pretty easily doing it this way – higher-mileage months may show up a particular weakness, or you may see common factors emerging – is it always the same side? Are the niggles coming when you are doing a particular type of workout or wearing a particular pair of shoes? Tracking in this way should throw up some red flags to keep an eye on.

LIFESTYLE: PRESSURES AND PITFALLS

In the midpack, you can do everything in your power to get your whole body health right. You're training better than ever, you're getting your rest and recovery right, you're even nailing down that strength stuff you've been putting off for the last couple of years, and reflecting on the process. Sometimes it's life that just has the habit of unpredictably getting in the way. Life regularly throws in curve balls, spanners (sometimes full-blown toolsets!), pressure points, unexpected trials and obstacles to navigate in, through and around. It's at this time that priorities, perspective and response are really important.

It really is just running.

Your priorities are going to change frequently during your time in the midpack. You're going to have pinch points, from work, family and things that land on you out of nowhere: illness, upheaval, bereavement. It's about how you react to these events that you have no or very little control over. It's about remembering the 'runner', who you really are, what you're about and why you run. Gaining some perspective over why you want to run, or why you even started, is really helpful.

Everyone, even the people at the top of their game, has an individual kind of pressure point and again that varies from person to person in and out of the midpack. We all have stress buttons that get pressed on a day-to-day basis and require us to respond in a healthy way. You've already seen our section on confidence and emotion regulation in Chapter 2. Running shouldn't be an extra thing that you have to 'do' or have on your list of stresses. It's up to you to recognise when running is no longer a positive enabler in your life. When you feel stretched, pushed, prodded, poked, dropped, helpless, overwhelmed, then cracking your running can be the glue that holds the rest of your well-being together. But it can also be the way in which you come unstuck. It's imperative as you move through the midpack that you learn how to harness the sticky sense of purpose and super strength of running rather than letting any anxiety, guilt or running pressure get on top of you. Very simply put, your running is important to you, and we recognise that (otherwise you wouldn't be reading this book) but please notice the times when your running needs to serve you differently. When you need to dial it back, reduce or even stop it for a while to enable you to focus with laser-sharp, unflustered focus on whatever is more pressing in your life at that particular moment. The ideal here is that you can use your running to continue to keep you balanced, healthy, strong and able to cope rather that pushing your limits, eroding your ability to face your everyday life, declining your performance and negatively impacting your overall wellness.

Stress buttons – what pushes yours and how running helps

Stress is one of the biggest drains on our overall well-being. It drives hormone changes in our body that shouldn't be sustained long term, and it often stops us exercising, eating well, sleeping well and having a positive lifestyle. Many of us use running when we're stressed to help clear our heads and reduce feelings of anxiety and it's been proven to help. What's more, the long-term benefits are becoming evident, too; some studies have shown that exercise can mitigate the negative impact of long-term stress. While these studies are still in their early stages, reducing your stress in the day-to-day will certainly leave you in a better state of well-being, and if running and exercise is the path to doing this, then that's a good thing.

The following are the major causes of stress:

- Work – hours, deadlines, promotion, long days, travel, dealing with people, losing work, events, social pressure.
- Family – responsibility, kids, money, holidays, time, illness, caring for others, loneliness.
- General crap in life – money, illness, life admin, car trouble, others' expectations.

Look at all of the stress buttons or triggers above and really recognise the ones that apply to you. Some of them will be constant, some will be occasional, it's very unusual if any of them draw a 'never'. The only thing even the greatest control freak can control when it comes to these factors is how you respond to them. Some of your stress buttons might respond very well to 'obviously, I can go running to cope with that'. You might be someone who can beautifully translate an argument with your boss (or your partner) to a tough run, but it's unlikely you can solve a money issue by booking a trip to go and do a race in a different country. It's how you respond to stress that should allow you to continue to keep running as a positive.

Shift happens

Working shifts can be disruptive. It's enough of a juggling act as it is with life, work and kids, without having to add into the mix long shift patterns that disrupt any kind of sleep and general routine. Runners who work shifts will have to constantly change their training routines, and will have to bear this in mind when planning and booking races, too. If shift work is new to you, or indeed if structured training is, you need to spend at least a couple of weeks working out how that's going to fit for you. You may be the kind of runner who likes to come off a long shift and go running straight away, regardless of the time; someone who prefers to run before work, again paying no attention to the time; or you could be someone who just can't fit running in when you are in a particular shift pattern. The latter would require a completely different structure of training to most 'standard' running plans. It's back to being personal again! You need to understand exactly how this works for you so that you can make progress, gain fitness and truly love the process of getting it all done. Keep in mind that a training plan doesn't have to just be a week at a time – other cycles may be better for your circumstances.

Lifestyle and how you react to it

This is the complicated pillar as it includes elements of all the others. Lifestyle choices are broad and varied, and so they should be, we're not robots. Yet the lifestyle choices we make have a short-, medium- and long-term impact on our current and future health status. What we do, with whom, how and when, our social connectedness, community relationships, economic stability, late nights, stressful days, missed meals, unhappy relationships, loneliness, isolation, sense of purpose and feeling of fulfilment all impact our overall well-being. The key is recognising what's important – what brings you joy and wellness – and ensuring those areas are protected.

Having a busy lifestyle is likely to be one of the biggest factors that affect your running. Everything we have mentioned so far in this chapter is in some way related to this. It's about the stresses and demands that come into play from work, from your family, how you sleep, whether you get to rest, how you train and sometimes how you respond to your body breaking down a little bit. Everyone in the midpack has stresses, some of which are out of their control, and it's how you react to them that matters. We mentioned earlier that you should try really hard to make sure you are 'using' your running in a relentlessly positive way. Escaping stress can be a way that running can support you. Placing these stresses on hold with a run in the great outdoors, to beautiful places in fresh air and nature, can help you regulate and manage difficult and uncomfortable situations. It gives you space to think of solutions and strategies, and sometimes simply to get away. Being free like this is the greatest of all running pleasures and it doesn't cost you anything.

There are going to be lifestyle factors that pose a threat to you running well and making progress as you move in the midpack. We won't go so far as to say you need to address your hedonistic rock-and-roll lifestyle because you already know that drink and drugs won't cut it on race day. It's sneaky lifestyle stuff that poses the most risk over time, such as how long you spend driving to work each day, your exposure to germs that might make you ill, a pre-existing health condition, even how much of your day is spent sitting at a desk; it's no good doing the latter and then at the end of it expecting to be able to throw your trainers on and kick like Kipchoge. So think outside the box and list the factors you have in your lifestyle that are potentially road-blocking your progress in the midpack. How many of them can you change or control? It's really not worth getting hung up on things you can't change and this could be a good exercise instead in learning which stresses you need to let go of. Go back to what we have said about how you respond to injury; your second response is usually much better for you than the first one.

You don't have to get your monk on

We're not telling you to reduce your risks by completely cutting out everything you enjoy. You probably have some experience by now of what it's like to run with a hangover or attempting to race having eaten something completely unsuitable the night before. What's generally more beneficial for us in the midpack, rather than completely cutting out the fun things, is to integrate them proportionately, manageably and appropriately into your life. Understand when they work and when they don't. There shouldn't be any guilt tied to celebrating or catching up with friends and loved ones with a few drinks – it should be a source of joy you look forward to, as you can be you, and not just you the runner. Allowing yourself the things you love in balance with great running will reduce stress, raise the happy hormones and probably make you a nicer person to be around. Whether it's a big night out or a great night in, plan for perfect timing if you can. It's usually worth it.

INJURY AND ENFORCED REST

At some time or another, and often more frequently than we would like, midpack runners are going to get injured. We are going to get anything from acute injuries such as a broken bone from slipping on ice or misjudging a landing in a cross-country run, to chronic injuries such as plantar fasciitis (we all know someone battling this, right?!), Achilles tendinopathy and even arthritic knees. We are probably most likely to recognise the overuse injuries such as responses or fractures, torn muscles, shin splints and the one-size-fits-all 'runner's knee'. These are the injuries we have a tendency to foolishly ignore for as long as is humanly possible, limping through everyday life and expecting to switch off the pain as soon as we put our trainers on.

Running injuries happen to us for a variety of reasons. We might be predisposed to something, we're not stretching enough or at all. We're not doing the right strength work, we're overloading, we're overtraining, we're not warming up, we're not cooling down and more generally sometimes we are just terribly bloody unlucky.

It's up to you to do what you can to avoid injury – hopefully you have some ideas now of how to do this – and to respond to it in an appropriate way if it happens. We are going to get into your history and approach to running in the next chapter and that's going to get you thinking about what has changed or not changed in your running in the time you've been in the midpack. You might be able to see where, if you're getting injured a lot, you can make some adjustments to your training to try to avoid it.

Running when you are injured is not the same thing as getting in the 'hurt locker' (*see* p. 179) and being uncomfortable when you're running hard. You can't avoid an injury by simply just ignoring it. It's not helpful to push through because you've got a race coming up. Running injured doesn't make you tough or bring you any sort of kudos. Getting injured costs you time out, money on physio and makes you a pain in the arse to be around. Let's be completely clear: we aren't physiotherapists and neither of us have any medical background so it's worth remembering that you're going to need the help of a professional if you find yourself feeling busted. In the midpack, we aren't usually blessed with having a 'team' around us like the elites have, but given how dedicated you are to running, you may already know who's good to call on in an injury crisis.

Recognise and react

Keeping a note in your training diary of regular niggles helps prevent injuries, as does patience and caution.

If you feel a niggle isn't improving with rest or if you have something that just keeps coming back, it's time to speak to a professional. Niggles should settle with some time off, and you definitely shouldn't be running if something happens that causes you to come to a complete stop. If you've ever felt the gunshot effect of a calf tearing you'll know what we mean. We can't tell you this enough: don't ask the internet for advice. Not only are your social media followers very unlikely to be professionals, but their experiences of injury will also vary widely. Get some recommendations for some great physios – especially those who specialise in running – and then switch your notifications off. Your starting point should be an accurate diagnosis from a qualified specialist.

We totally understand how being injured feels and the frustration it brings. Injury can at best give you a much-needed enforced rest for tired legs and at worst completely disengage you from your friends and your healthy routines. You might start by reacting emotionally, catastrophising and going immediately to worst-case scenario. You might think things like: 'I can't believe this has happened again!', 'I have wasted all that training!', 'This has cost me X amount of weeks and X amount of money in the races I have booked'. It's much better to show yourself a bit of patience, see what your physio says, then go to a new 'first' reaction, something like: 'I have a plan to help this heal', 'I can do X instead', even perhaps eventually the dizzy heights of 'This might make me a better runner in the long term'.

Staying connected during periods of injury is really important to your mental and emotional well-being. It's understandable that you don't want to go to races and hold your friends' bags while they race around experiencing everything you are missing, and we know it's hard seeing everyone's training runs popping up on social media (especially if they are complaining about it). Some withdraw from the community completely, and that's OK if that's all that will help you through it, but some positive steps instead might be to volunteer at races or at parkrun, hit the unfollow button temporarily on social media and, basically, don't go bonkers doing loads of other stuff instead that you a) don't enjoy and b) will make you feel just as broken. We see runners regularly taking to other forms of exercise and going nuts with it, making injuries even worse, rather than backing off completely. Good physiotherapists will have a plan of action for you and will have the best ideas for cross-training that will help you to retain fitness and return to running as soon as it's safe to do so.

Most importantly, stop beating yourself up

Just be kind to yourself. If you're injured, you need to give yourself a break. Your reaction to injury is vital in how you eventually respond and heal.

Use the time to do stuff that's good for you and don't feel guilty about it. Use your support networks, things you enjoy doing and nature as the best ways to heal.

The hardest bit about returning from injury is acting with caution. You're going to need patience and that's often not our strong point. We shudder when we see long, fast 'out testing the...' runs on Strava, which run the risk of knocking you straight back to the acute stage of your injury. Walking longer with occasional short spells of running that you can progress (e.g. two minutes of slow jogging, twice in one walk one day, wait a few days then repeat with three minutes if you have no pain) is a great way to make sure your body is ready to jog, and then to run. It's much better to find your return to running tedious but pain-free rather than putting yourself out of action for another two or three weeks just by rushing back.

FEMALE HEALTH AND CYCLES

Talking about your cycle isn't and shouldn't be a taboo. For women who have a regular 'normal' cycle, it's going to make a difference to your running, how you feel and how you train at various times of every month. We recommend downloading a tracking app as a starting point if you haven't already done so – tracking your cycle between the menstrual, follicular, ovulation, and luteal phases is a good place to start. Anji found that tracking cycle days and symptoms during them was a game changer during a big cycle of marathon training and helped to explain why some weeks things just didn't seem to click while others felt easy and she could be physically challenged more.

Tracking shows quickly how your body changes and feels through each phase, how long the phases are, and tracking these changes and symptoms is extremely worthwhile. Your body is going to change within the phases in many ways, including your body temperature, metabolism and mood, before we even start on how you feel during your period. Dr Georgie Bruinvels and Dr Jess Piasecki are dedicated in their work with female athletes and their health, and both agree tracking is the most worthwhile place to start. Both athletes themselves, Georgie and Jess recommend finding out more as an individual and being prepared to look into how you fuel, plan training load, manage stress, sleep and maintain routine according to your cycle.

Everyone is different and factors will come into play, such as whether you're taking the contraceptive pill, how old you are, any health conditions you have and what your nutrition looks like, but there are likely to be a couple of things that line up for you. The key thing is that if you get a handle on phases of your cycle and when to expect them, you can arrange your training to get the best from yourself. It's a worthwhile way of starting to plan effective training.

BE GOOD TO YOURSELF

Your goal as a midpack runner should be to find joy in the running that you do regularly and when we put it like that it's quite simple. We know that finding that joy can at times be a bit of a puzzle, but it's worth taking the steps to get it just right. You should be able to flex between lifestyle pressures, stress buttons and triggers, avoid injury and keep everything balanced – all

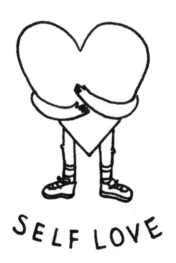

Be good to yourself

SELF LOVE

of which is the best route to cultivating your progress. This is really all about you. Your relationships, your overall health and happiness are what create your overall health and wellness, and building your running on top of that should make it a very easy puzzle to solve. Spend some time reflecting on this chapter, especially the sections on stress buttons and bullet-proofing, and hopefully you'll never need to return to our section on injury or getting back from it.

Be good to yourself, be reflective, be kind to yourself and the rest should follow.

It's time to start looking at training.

FOUR

TRAINING

A BLEND OF ART AND APPLICATION

Training is much more than simply the hard work that needs to be done for you to run better.

Let's get deep! What gives you purpose? What gives you direction? What supports your fulfilment? What fuels your passions? What ignites your ambition? What makes you feel great? What drives your training also brings meaning, purpose, fulfilment and direction to your running. It's important to see it like that, otherwise there's a danger you'll regard your training simply as something functional, something you have to do, something performance focused that gets you where want to go, period. Yes, for sure it does that, and it's needed to do that, yet it does so much more. You're reading this book because you want to move through the midpack but also because you want to enjoy your running, you want to allow it to bring joy to your life, to encourage and nourish you and to help you construct and maintain your running life and self. When you see training as more than the functional specifics, more than the science, more than the physiology and more than the outcomes, when you see training more about creativity, energy, purpose and progress and when you focus on the process of your training, you are setting yourself up for a more lifelong, life-enhancing love of training and of running that also helps you to achieve the moving-in-the-midpack goals you're looking for.

Training is what ties together your goals, actions and aspirations with what you actually do. Training should give your running direction, strategy and purpose, and you should do it with passion, devotion, energy and determination. Whether you're a regular runner who gets off on the buzz of training in a group, or a self-motivated lone wolf, training is what you have to want to do (most of the time at least!) to make sure you're going to make the kind of progress that you want to make in the ways in which you want to make it. We've harped on a bit about process so far, and this chapter is all about the process you're going to engage in.

We are going to go through some of the principles behind the science of training, what it is and why you have to do it. We're going to give you ideas and a bit of background on why it matters, and we are going to pull it all together to help you frame your goals, work towards your targets, and give you some real practical tools to go and get them.

We are going to guide you through making decisions on what to train for and how to actively engage with the process. We will look at the real fundamentals of training. We are going to help you to navigate and understand progression, load, specificity, recovery, frequency (and we are going to show you that they are much less scary than they sound). We are going to talk about 'training pillars' and how to get the balancing of them right, and we are going to show you some of our favourite workouts, which might help to bring some variety to your running. We are going to look at the concepts of the 'dickhead button' and the 'hurt locker' and we are going to get you excited about planning your next big block of training.

We're not here to make this complicated. We are going to do our best to filter out the noise and cut through the fancy language that isn't really necessary for you to build your training purposefully. There's a lot of fluff out there that won't do you any favours, so we are going to keep it direct: to get better and to move in the midpack, you have to train.

To achieve a target, you have to prepare yourself accordingly – having unrealistic expectations based on what you have and have not done is a sure way to lose enjoyment in your running. Put plainly, training will make race day better, more pleasurable, more likely to have a great outcome. Think in the long game of good process leading to good outcome. Training gives us better engines, creates efficiency, makes us better.

Training is the act of participating in regular, structured running that is planned and purposeful. It's intentional, sustainable, progressive, appropriate, involves overload, specificity, flexibility, adaptation, cultivation, curiosity and commitment. Training can be done for many different reasons: it can be to define a specific personal challenge, run a distance or a pace or reach a place, target a particular event, or define specific individual milestones you'd like reach. We'd encourage you to actively take real ownership of setting out that purposeful journey. What does it mean to you? Why do you want to do it? What can you do to get there? When you've got your eyes on the prize – that run goal – effective training is empowering, enabling and loaded! Training is all about the what, the when and the how of your running. Let's get it on!

START BY LOOKING AT YOUR FOUNDATIONS

Training is supposed to be executed to make you a 'better' runner, not break you down. It's supposed to hurt, but not ruin you. It's supposed to stretch you, but not damage you. It's about knowing when to turn it up and when to dial it down. Without doubt the most important thing to reflect on before reviewing, planning, designing and implementing training is the status of your foundation. You simply can't train meaningfully, properly or effectively from an uneven kick-off. Making the decision to commit to your training is a super-positive step, and one that you shouldn't take lightly. We want you to spend some time now thinking about the foundations, the training pillars, you're going to build on.

You found out more about your personal foundation in the previous chapter, and you should have a good understanding now about what is likely to affect your training in your day-to-day life. Without stable foundations (and a little wobble room!) you can't have strong pillars. Without strong pillars, fundamentals of training (the stuff you have to actually knuckle down and deliver on), such as building blocks, can be hard to establish. Our foundations are the really important bricks at the core of us: our work, our health, general life stuff and our family. At any time, something in your foundation might not be quite right but it's how you adapt and adjust to stresses that allows you to keep on progressing. Your training pillars are going to sit on top of that.

Training pillars

Your training pillars are rest (and sleep), nutrition, emotional state, and the types of training you do. That includes the consistency, frequency and time spent doing it. Can you see you're asking a lot of yourself if those foundations of 'you' are a bit wobbly? We are all, at least some of the time, winging it for at least one of them. You are likely to be wrestling through some kind of internal wobble at any given time. We aren't saying you can't get anything from the process of your training if it isn't 100 per cent right. We just want you to really think about how you can make the pillars of training work for you. Lots of this is actually in your control. You will get some pinch points at any given time that may start to feel destructive, but we want you to be able to recognise them and change or adapt what you can. A great foundational training question to ask yourself when planning and before every workout is: 'How is this run making me a better runner and contributing towards where I want my running to go?'

Training and the types of training are the last important piece of the puzzle. This chapter is going to walk you through getting a good handle on all the elements that will help you to get from where you are to where you want to be, with some great process along the way. It's not only one foot in front of the other, and getting that right can lead you to the satisfaction of achieving something you've worked damned hard for.

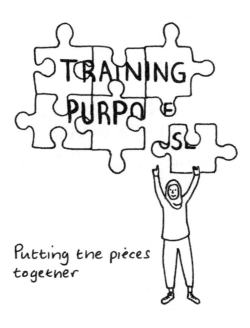

Putting the pieces
together

DEFINING YOUR TRAINING PURPOSE

What's the point of training? Why bother? What's it all about? What's got your attention? What do you want to run, where and why? Goals and aspirations in the running midpack can go anywhere from running the fastest mile you've ever run, qualifying for your dream overseas race or running a distance you've never done before, in a time you've never done before, to the joy of completing something you've heard so much about from others, or taking part in a type of race over a terrain that's out of your comfort zone.

While aspirations in the midpack will vary massively, the process of going and getting them via some focused, structured and purposeful running looks very similar. Remember that a goal should be something for you that is motivating, inspiring, challenging, different and exciting. Goals should be personal, meaningful to you, and the process of chasing them should be one you want to be a part of. Take the time to decide what yours could look like and how long it will take you to achieve. Then decide what that commitment looks like and do it. Think of it along the lines of your personal training budget. Consider how much time, energy, effort and motivation you're willing to invest in committing to your goal. Be realistic about your time. Don't overcommit or be overambitious. Seek balance and a fruitful return. There is no scope for 'if', 'but' or 'maybe' here. Your commitment to your goal is your pledge to yourself that you are going to make the required, and your desired, effort to reach your personal aspirations.

DEFINING YOUR 'BIG ONE': BIG GOALS, LITTLE GOALS, CARDBOARD BOX GOALS

How do you decide how important your race is? When setting your race aspiration, it helps to prioritise it in your mind. How important the race is to you shapes your approach to running it.

A race

It's a big goal. It means a lot. You've been prepping for months. It's really hard to get into. It's a proper lifetime goal to complete. A real physical, emotional and financial (?) investment. It really does matter! You might be chasing a personal best, targeting an emotional and physical summit, laying it all out there to lifetime achieve something.

B race

Little goal. It's important, but not a deal-breaker. Often, these races are to gauge fitness, to practise routines, paces, to gain experience. They are still relevant but as you're driven by process anyway you're not too miffed if these races don't quite work out as well as you'd planned or hoped. There is always something to learn and benefit from in a B race. You'll probably have more of these in your race planning pocket than A races.

C race

Cardboard box goal. These events are the floor-fillers of your race calendar. They are less significant, low-key, journey races, ones where you might prioritise a social catch-up over a speed round.

DON'T JUST THINK ABOUT IT

A lot goes into choosing what events you'd like to do, and even more should go into getting ready for them. Once you've identified the what and the why of your racing, it's time to get real about the how. This is the point at which understanding yourself and what works for you really helps. We see loads of midpack runners going for the route of randomly searching online and trawling through the myriad of 'training advice' but it's really important to understand that the best way to help you reach your personal aspirations is to be driven by you. Getting to know what makes you tick, how to adapt, what makes you twitchy and how you respond, all relates to the way in which your training will work. This takes a bit more time, effort and experience and a willingness to fail (a few times!), learn, adapt and grow in your running. We are going to help.

Bring in the balance

Having the 'why' is a key place to start but we want you to go deeper than that. Some midpack runners will have run for many years and made little progress, and that's a good time to look at a deeper why. What is your real starting point? What is your history of training? Look at how you have approached training in the past – did you have the balance right between training and recovering, for example? Everyone has a different starting point. If you've suffered from a series of very similar injuries over the years, that's something you should start by addressing. If your mindset is fixed, negative or you're wrestling with confidence issues, go back to Chapter 2 and work through some of those ideas, too. It's all part of your wider, more comprehensive, personalised approach to training.

The best way to get the results you're after and train how you want to train is to take responsibility for planning your own running schedule. After all, you know yourself as a runner better than anyone else. You are a great coach to yourself, you might just need a little support, advice and scaffolding around you to help you realise that. A good self-written training plan includes all the ingredients you want in your training in the right quantities and at the right times. The key with writing your own plan is that it is personal to you, lets you take ownership of your running and empowers you to execute the plan. Runners train in different ways and there is no single 'right way'. What works for one runner might not work for another. One person's 'easy' run is another's 'steady' or 'threshold' pace. This is especially true in the midpack, with our mixture of backgrounds, experience, goals and aspirations. In planning your training, make sure it's designed with you in mind. It's all about you.

START WHERE YOU LEFT OFF

As an experienced midpack runner, you've been here before. If you keep doing what you've always done, in the same way you've always done it, don't be surprised if you keep getting what you've always got. Avoid the temptation of slipping quickly back into training comfort when beginning a new training focus or building block. It's important to consider your training background, your recent running history, what's worked and what's bombed, and what can be binned and built on before you leap into your next training cycle.

1. *Take time to reflect*

After a long season, a target race or at the end of your running year, it pays to review things properly. Building up to and executing a goal race can take it out of you and leave you feeling a little lost, so don't rush the reflection process. This helps your follow-up training phases. Instead of going out for another run and immediately slipping into what you already know and all the things you've done before, sit down and spend quality time intentionally thinking back over your performances and how they felt. A well thought-out review will help inform your future training and improve your racing.

It's always a good idea to write your review down. Try answering the following questions:

- What were the highlights of your running year?

  Think about the things that you were really proud of during the year. This could be your race results, personal achievements or other running-related success stories. Include anything and everything.

- What did you do in your i) training and ii) racing to achieve these highlights?

  Think about the things you did well in your training and racing. What worked for you? Be really specific. What did you do that you really feel contributed to your successes? Practical, logistical, physical, nutritional, psychological ... everything you can think of that you did that had a positive impact on your highlights. List as many positive things as you can, even the stuff that sounds irrelevant. Keep asking yourself 'what else did I do that worked?'

- What are the top five 'success behaviours' you are going to repeat?

  These are the top actions drawn from above that worked and that you are going to keep in your training regime and racing routines. These are your personal success ingredients. The things you want to keep doing to keep improving, enjoying your running and building on your successes. These should be all about you and focused on the process.

- What would you like to do differently or get better at in your i) training and ii) racing?

  Think about the things that didn't go too well for you. The gaps, omissions and things you'd have changed or done differently. This might be mistakes you made in training or things you got wrong in racing. Did you do as much preparation as you'd have liked? Did you eat as healthily as you'd hoped? Did you crack under the pressure in your big race? What were some of the reasons for this? What didn't go well? Why didn't it go well? Again, keep asking yourself for more. You're going to ask yourself some difficult questions here and it pays to be honest.

- What are your top five priority areas for future success?

  Decide and define what you want successful running to look like for you. Is it about running faster times, running longer, doing more (or fewer races), experiencing new things in running, setting personal process targets, or realising another running ambition? From the things you identified that you'd like to do differently, what would you like to change the most? In order of priority to you, list the things that you'd most like to do in your running next year that will help you improve and be a success. For example: i) I'd like to be more consistent in my running; ii) I'd like to focus more on fuelling better.

- What are the barriers/obstacles that exist?

  Next, think about the barriers that you need to overcome to work towards these priorities. For example, what stops you from being more consistent in your running? Illness, injury, work commitments, social life, lack of time? What help and support do you need from other people to help you in this area?

- What are you going to do about it and when?

  Next to each priority area, write down one clear action that you can take. Something that you can take control of and do that will contribute towards overcoming barriers and turning your problem areas into progress. Include a date, signalling when you are going to start putting this action in place. For example: 'To be more consistent in my running I am going to protect my time to run by going out to run before work on two out of three mornings each week.'

2. Think about your aspirations

When planning any training, it's vital to consider your aspirations once you've been through your reflections. What do you want your training plan to help you achieve? Are you aiming at a specific event, personal challenge or race in the future? Is it far enough away to be achievable? How far away from this goal do you feel you are right now? Really focusing in tightly on what you want to achieve helps you to clearly structure your planning towards it. Think back to the goal and focus more now on the what than the why.

3. What is your training budget?

Establish from the outset how much time you can realistically give to your training each week (in hours, workout opportunity frequency, or both) and how many weeks you feel you are able to commit at this level. Look at your current work, social, home and lifestyle schedule and determine how much time you have available to train. For everyone in the midpack, this varies massively. Often, we see people at the start of a training cycle overbudgeting because they're so keen to crack on, without being honest about how that's going to feel a few weeks down the line. Devise a structure that is realistic rather than overambitious and involve the people closest to you so they can help you to see if it's going to be a struggle. It's far better to undercommit and consistently overdeliver in your training than to overcommit and keep dropping workouts, get frustrated and end up losing your mojo and packing it all in. Underpromise, overdeliver, every time.

It may take a number of weeks to establish and integrate your budget with your commitments and other priorities, but developing a routine and forming a habit is a great place to start.

Here are some key questions to consider when you're planning:

1. How many times a week are you going to run? Three, four, five?
2. How long can you allocate for each workout? 40 minutes, 60 minutes, 90 minutes? Think also about where in the day it will fit in.
3. Where is each workout taking place? From home, from work?
4. Who is the workout with? A club/group, solo?
5. What other things do you want to include? Time to stretch, trips to the physio, strength and/or conditioning, cross-training? When will you include these?

When developing your routine, determine the best time for you to run that doesn't compromise your work or family commitments. Is this three times a week before work, at lunchtime or four times a week in the evenings, or a combination? Short, time-efficient runs in the week and longer runs at the weekend? Get your routine planned out, then get specific and determine what you're going to do and when. We talked a lot about your stress buttons in the section on lifestyle pressure in Chapter 3, and making sure your planned routine doesn't cause any of these buttons to be pressed is really important for your emotional state, as well as your relationships – the true basis of you.

TRAINING FUNDAMENTALS: THE PRINCIPLES OF EVERY GOOD TRAINING JOURNEY

It can be tricky to remember all the elements required to build into a plan to make it work for you. There's a lot to think about. When you've been running a long time, you might even find some things, such as progression, consistency and load, come naturally to you. You kick your season prep off in a particular way, you've got your routes, your paces and your groups, you slot almost effortlessly into it. If you want to move in the midpack, though, it pays to remind yourself of fundamentals such as specificity, progression, consistency, overload, reversibility and recovery, and freshen (and possibly shift) your thinking about the importance of how they integrate into your running plan. The best personal training planning comes when you understand these fundamentals but you also understand, through experience and theory, through practice, trial and retrial how these things work for you.

Every training plan is going to include some of the same things to make you a better runner and guide you to successfully reaching your goals. These are the most important.

Specificity

Train in the way in which you wish to race and to prepare for the specific demands of the event in which you are running. If you get specifics wrong you'll end up bowling into your big day lacking all the right tools you need to do the job properly. Training without the specifics, or failing to understand the real demands of your event, and how you might develop these and then how you might respond to them in training, is an almost certain way to flunk race day. It's like preparing for your biggest exam – but spending your time learning and revising all the wrong material. Getting the specifics right means drawing upon the knowledge of others, the knowledge of the event and your knowledge of yourself. When you do that then you'll have no real surprises on race day. It's in the bag!

Lukewarm and wishy-washy is no good if you aspire to see training progress and results realised in performances. You know by now that you can't prepare for a long-distance mountain running event if all you're doing in training is short reps on a flat surface. Specificity in training is easier if you've been specific in your goals, so make sure that's your true starting point when you are planning. Let's really look at what you're going to be challenged by when it comes to that goal event, and make that your focus. You need to consider when you plan your training how many miles you need to cover each week, how many hard effort sessions you'll really need to put in to make progress. To put it simply: you're unlikely to achieve a specific outcome goal (for example, hold a sustained target pace) if you don't do any running at that pace in practice, and you're not going to be able to run as long at that pace if you don't build up to it over time.

Overload

Overload shouldn't sound like a scary term. Overload in training is really just about adapting to doing something more. Whether you're running more, lifting heavier weights, jumping higher, learning a new skill, you're overloading your body or mind. You're asking yourself to do some things you're not used to, and that's OK. It's nothing to be scared of. It's important. Overloading is basically adaptation, changing your body and improving your fitness to cope with what you want it to do. Training, overloading and adapting is what is going to make you run faster, or further, over a new terrain, and make you more comfortable on race day when you ask it to. Training and overloading (adding 'load' and building progress) challenges us by asking a little more each time, week on week. It will not only give you confidence, but it will also physically change you, too. The process of doing this gradually is what makes you fitter and stronger, leading to more adaptation and progress in your running when it pays off.

Overload means doing a little more running, putting in a little more effort, pushing your boundaries a little further as you get fitter and stronger. If you just did the same type of running all the time then you would see initial improvements but then you'd plateau and not get much better as time progressed. You'd probably also get pretty bored! It is through overloading your body that it learns to deal with the pressure you place it under and over time adapts so that subsequent workouts feel easier. You can overload your running by adding more distance (increasing the duration/volume), running more often (increasing the frequency/volume), and running faster (increasing the intensity), as well as by changing the type of running that you do. Of course, you cannot simply keep overloading your system by running more and more and faster and faster or you'll break down.

With careful overloading, which is planned and includes time for you to recover properly between your runs, you feel yourself starting to adapt – that's where some of the magic starts to happen. Your watch might inform you that you are hitting a higher VO_2 max (*see* p. 111), have a good training status, you'll see messages popping up on Strava to tell you that a familiar route is now 'trending faster'. You might find your weekly trot around parkrun is getting faster without you really putting much extra effort in, or you're overtaking people in your group who are usually ahead of you. Adaptation is cool because the workouts that used to hurt before don't hurt quite as much and you can get further or faster before the Tuesday legs* hit. You're adapting, you're progressing and that's one of the best feelings in the process of training.

*Tuesday legs: The day-two-after-run pain experienced by runners, which is difficult to describe to others. The period during which soreness, lethargy and heaviness in the legs is difficult to ignore, especially when going up and down stairs or getting up from or going down into a seated position.

It's really important that your overload is carefully linked to your training goal. Some runners will look for successes in the form of smaller stepping-stone goals along the way to their main target, and mini overloads towards these can cause some burnout that isn't necessary. Staying focused on the process of the training with overload that is specific to the end goal is far more enjoyable than burning out halfway through a cycle of training while you try to PB everything along the way.

Consistency

Probably the most important fundamental of any training is consistency. It's the single most relevant thing that will shift your performance. Keep on showing up. If you're finding something hard, it probably means you need to do it more, or do it in a different way. Being consistent in your training is something you can't overlook. Engaging in regular training that allows you to grow and adapt has a great pay-off and links a lot to how confident you feel in your running, too. Looking back over a bank of progressive, great workouts that get longer or faster can give you the reassurance that you're getting closer to your goal. It feels wonderful to look back at all those ticked-off sessions in your plan. Consistency is everyone's secret weapon in the midpack.

Consistency has to be there to get your training right. Consistency of getting out and running regularly helps you to build routine, prepares your body and mind for what you are frequently asking it to do, and helps you to build week on week on week on your achievements.

However, it isn't about consistently getting out and smashing yourself to bits. Blowing your legs to pieces every time you run may look super impressive on Strava but it's not going to provide you with good experience in the long term. Being overzealous doesn't help. Being cautiously ambitious does. Make sure you are allowing time to run slower, to recover, to just run. It's been well documented that marathon world record holder Eliud Kipchoge runs his recovery sessions at slower than 8 minutes/mile (5 minutes/km) pace. If he can slow down by more than 3 minutes/mile (1 minute 52 seconds/km), then you can, too. Taking care in your training to hit hard workouts when they are planned and have purpose rather than pushing yourself to do it hard every single time can also help you to avoid injury.

We think this quote from coach Dan Robinson, an expert in exercise physiology and fatigue, nails it: 'Slightly conservative but consistent training will bring about greater improvement than more aggressive but sporadic sessions. Perhaps most crucially training in a more measured way significantly reduces the risk of injury, the bane of a runner's life and the biggest single hindrance to progress.'

That said, if all you did were be 'super consistent' you'd always stay the same runner you've always been. You want to settle for mediocrity? Then keep doing your mediocre training year in year out. Train the same, stay the same. It's healthy to ramp it up, but at the same time you have to be super confident about how much, when.

Progression

Progression is very closely related to overload and is especially important when you look closely at your training. Progression means very gradually increasing the amount of running, faster running or longer-distance running that you engage in. This progression doesn't take place all at once, rather over a prolonged period of time. Every good training programme allows you to build up over time to your goal distance or pace, allowing breaks when you can back off and recover, too. To a certain extent, progression also seems to happen naturally. As you get fitter, stronger and more accustomed to running you'll want to run further, for longer and faster! But remember, a key feature of getting progression right is not to increase the quantity (frequency and duration) and the quality (how fast you run) of your workouts at the same time. Good progression is balanced, seamless and smooth.

A general rule you will have seen, particularly when training for longer distance, is to never increase your long run distance by more than 10 per cent each week, but it's important to also include some 'backing off' weeks when you reduce your training to allow some planned recovery, too. Recovering well is part of the process that allows you to progress further.

Something we really want you to think about as you move through your training is that progression is rarely a completely linear process.

Principles of progress

- Be patient. You'll probably want progress to happen faster than it actually will. There is a lag in terms of physiological development and adaptation or benefits to training. This means you'll do it, but you won't feel any benefits for a while. In fact, while juggling load you'll probably feel worse before you notice any improvement and start to feel better.

- Be flexible. Progression won't always go to plan. Expect this and allow some freedom and movement for a few blips. Being flexible means you can roll with the punches that training throws at you and you don't throw your toys out of pram when it doesn't go entirely as you'd hoped. Sometimes you'll need to switch things around, do less or bin something. Be alright with that.

- Be gradual. Go too fast, too soon and you'll bust. There's a real temptation when getting stuck into training to throw yourself into it. You're new, you're committed, you're fired up, you're intentional, motivated and coiled! The trouble is, get that build wrong because you're all excited and you risk snapping. It's OK to give yourself a decent training lead in (a base phase) and allow a shallow progress curve.

- Be appropriate. You don't suddenly become a different runner. It takes time to allow progress and deep change in your running to happen. If you're doing things differently, trying a new training approach, a different event, do it appropriately. Appropriately for you, and for your running aspirations.

- Be contextual. Here we mean understand your context and situation. Progress only works if you do it within an environment that promotes progress. If you're constantly hitting barriers (these could be fatigue, child care, relationships, work) then you've underestimated the power, relevance and significance of your context and are setting yourself up for progress failure.

- Be careful. Give yourself a chance! So often we see runners who simply neglect the basics and keep the hammer down and keep pushing. This isn't effective. Period.

Reversibility (it's all too easy to lose it fast)

Despite what your mind might tell you, you're not going to lose all your fitness in a matter of a couple of days or due to occasional missed runs. Keeping a regular, purposeful, process-focused routine means you are gaining that fitness all the time and having a few days off when life gets in the way, you're not feeling great, not sleeping well or you're resting a niggle isn't going to make that much of a difference. There are times when midpack runners might forget this, and being so focused on the goal and a little fear of losing the fitness means they are tempted to run through the things that signal they probably need a break. We will come to the dickhead button soon.

You probably think that if you stop running, you'll lose your fitness quickly. In reality, you're not going to reverse all your hard work in a few days like that. However, it's worth remembering that as a general rule missing one week's training *does* require three weeks of effort to get back to the same level. It doesn't matter if you miss a few runs – when you pick it up next time you probably won't notice – but make a habit of it and you'll certainly find that your fitness level and running ability have dropped. The longer you stop doing it for, the longer it takes to get your fitness back. In this case, it's about not panicking if you end up missing some runs. You need to resist the urge to rush back after a lay-off. Take your time to re-adapt; rebuild your running through engaging in a planned and progressive road back to fitness with one eye always on process.

Recovery

This is explicitly linked to progression and overload and is probably the most crucial but at the same time the most neglected training principle. Recovery is a hugely important element you need to think about in planning your running training. When you train hard, you overstress your body and the training benefit or effect comes after training when your body repairs and rebuilds stronger. Effective recovery takes place if you allow your body sufficient time to rest and refuel. The importance of sleep and diet in recovery shouldn't be underestimated. You cannot run hard every day.

UNDERSTANDING TYPES OF RUNNING

When you're putting the pieces together to roll out your training, a further fundamental to understand is what types of running to do, when to do them, how much of them to do, and how to do them! This is related to the specifics of your training outcomes and the particular benefits you're seeking. For example, if you want to run faster, but all you do in training is plod along at the same old pace, getting faster simply isn't going to happen. To understand what types of running to put in place and when, you need to know the demands of your personal challenge (e.g. a 5k PB, a faster marathon or your first ultra) and the relative amount of time, priority and focus you should be directing at different types of training.

Different running paces

Depending on how you arrived in the midpack, you might already have a lot of experience in running different types of 'sessions' and paces. Here are the key paces to consider in your training. Again, the balance and focus of these is relative and should be adjusted to the specifics of what you're actually training for.

Easy (less than 50 per cent effort)
To see improvement without breaking down you'll need some recovery runs. These should be nice and easy and you should feel relaxed. Enjoy the scenery.

101

You should be breathing easily and be capable of holding a conversation throughout the run. If you're a new/novice runner then you'll probably be questioning whether any runs feel easy and holding a conversation may feel impossible all of the time! Slow down, walk if necessary and control your effort. Easy running is where you start to build your endurance – that important part of running that makes you stronger at running for longer.

Steady (around 60 per cent effort)
These are the bread and butter of your training, the 'miles in the bank'. These steady runs build your aerobic base, which acts as the foundation for the rest of your training. Conversations are still possible at this pace but in sentences rather than a long gossip!

Tempo (around 70 per cent effort)
You're probably doing some tempo running without even realising that's what you should call it. Tempo is a step up from steady running and a step back from threshold. If we are going for percentages again, it's about 70 per cent effort and it's a pace you can hang on to for longer than that high-intensity stuff. We love tempo running that is sandwiched between other sessions, such as running easy for 50 minutes then into a faster-paced finish for the last 10. You can block tempo running into an easy longer run, too, and it works just as well in distance as it does in time. Upping the tempo, for example, in the middle 3 miles (4.8km) of a 10-miler (16km) can crank you up out of cruise control and get you working harder in a gear shift that just feels fun. Tempo is good for endurance and the more you do it, the more your perception of effort will change.

Threshold (feels like 80 per cent+ effort)
Running at 'threshold' pace is about running under 'controlled discomfort' and is great for improving your running economy. After the long endurance runs, threshold runs are probably your most valuable workouts. You will find them slightly uncomfortable and they'll require concentration, but they are well worth the effort. You'll only be capable of uttering a couple of words as you run. As you get fitter and more experienced, you'll learn how to find your

own 'threshold' pace and this will change the fitter, stronger and faster you get. You can get very specific pace guidance on your threshold if you venture into the world of lab testing – it's not just for the elites – but if that's not your thing, work on around 80 per cent of your max-out effort.

Fast (feels like 90 per cent+ effort)

This is the kind of burn-up pace you know right away you can't hold on to for long! It's high-intensity, short duration, uncomfortable, and super beneficial for boosting your top-end anaerobic capacity. When you run at this pace you can't keep it up for long, it hurts and your legs go wobbly after about 60 seconds (longer if you're trained at this stuff).

Different running types

Understanding the different ways of running really helps you to structure your planning and your paces. Not every run is the same, and not every run brings about the same benefits. Although it's not that complicated, if you want to increase speed, spend more time running fast; if you want to increase stamina, spend more time on your feet; if you want to increase speed endurance, spend increasing time somewhere in the middle. It also really benefits runners to truly understand both the spectrum of different paces but also the range of different ways in which they can incorporate these into a successful training plan.

Fartlek

Fartlek running is translated from the Swedish term 'speed play' and that's what we need to keep in mind – play is fun, fartlek is fun! Fartlek is great to do over varied terrain because it's fast, slow, whatever you feel like. Fartlek is best done with a variation of easy, steady and fast running for different times and distances with varying amounts of recovery.

Intervals

Interval running is more formal, structured speed work that is done at a high intensity. Intervals include repetitions of time or distance and are followed by periods of rest or recovery. Your intervals should be set at pace or effort; they're not times for conversation or chatting to catch up with friends. That said, some of you will get a lot out of running them in a group, in order to bring out a bit of good old-fashioned natural competition. Interval/ high-intensity running should require you to get into the hurt locker and get uncomfortable: hanging on in there is what will make you fitter and faster when it comes to race day. It's so important to learn to cope with the discomfort of the hurt locker over and over again to prepare your body for the test of racing.

Sustained effort

This type of run session is designed to help you learn to suffer in controlled discomfort for a while. A sustained effort run could last 30–90 minutes (depending on your goals) and sees you put yourself in a place at tempo-threshold pace for a sustained amount of time. It's not a sustained effort if you chat effortlessly to your mates while gliding along, neither is it a sustained effort if you smash it until the end of your road and run out of gas.

Distance

Long, slow distance runs. Long runs are vital for building your 'engine' and endurance, especially when you're working towards a longer-distance event. The term 'long run' is again subjective. Your long run in a marathon might be up to 23 miles (37km), while a long run to someone working towards their first 10km race (6.2 miles) could take them to 5 miles (8km) or upwards. We actually prefer to work in time, looking at how long you're going to spend on your feet, and we find this can offset some anxiety many people have about running further than they have before. Slow-paced long runs are often a midpack runner's favourite, being the most enjoyable way to catch up with friends and spend a Sunday morning.

Hills

You can 'do' hill running as a type of interval training or as part of a longer run. Hill reps can be measured in distance, time or number of uphill efforts. Depending on what you want to get out of your hill sessions, it's good to vary the gradient and length of the hill you're running. The idea is to maintain a hard effort up and jog back down again as you recover.

A note on warming up and cooling down

Warming up and cooling down should bookend your runs, especially when you're doing a workout such as an interval session. They're quite a personal thing that you will have learned over time, but it can take most people around 15 minutes to settle into a run before they can give it full beans, so build this into your budget for each workout. The same goes for a cool-down – a good 10–15 minutes at a very easy jog is great to shake out any tight muscles and reflect on the work you've just done. Warming up and cooling down isn't as important on your longer runs, and they don't need to come into recovery and easy runs at all.

TRAINING ZONES: HEART RATE AND EFFORT PERCEPTION – 'HOW DO YOU KNOW HOW HARD TO RUN?'

Have you ever been running with someone and they look down at their watch, read the screen, check their 'beats per minute' and ask you: 'What's your heart rate?' You glance down, puffing, and gasp back '162'. You're running together, so you're running at the same pace, but you most likely are not running at the same relative intensity. This is a really important thing when seeking to understand heart rate (HR). It's individual. It must be interpreted as *your* data. It simply won't be the same (although it might be similar) to someone else's. You are seeking to observe patterns and understand trends in your own heart rate data.

Heart rate shifts at different intensities can be indicative of fitness improvements (i.e. lower heart rate at higher intensity, lower average heart rate for sustained intensity, quicker return to resting heart rate) but also heart rate increases at rest or during exercise can be indicative of fatigue or illness. A word of caution: erratic or sudden fluctuations in heart rate could be related to something other than training and you should seek specialist advice if you experience these.

We're often asked about informing training using HR data and heart rate zones. HR training can show you how hard you can run in different workout or 'heart rate' zones (how fast your heart beats depending on how hard you're working) and it can be a brilliant tool for training. Depending on where you look, you will see HR zones defined in different ways, usually through five stages, where one is the easiest and five is the hardest you can go. Remember, it's very individual. The zones indicate changes to your personal heart rate and can be utilised to help guide your training intensity.

Typical training heart rate zones

1. Easy – low aerobic/ endurance/warm-up
   This is your easiest jogging, running very slowly and at easy conversational pace.
2. Steady – aerobic/moderate/easy
   This is still easy pace and should be something you're hitting in your long endurance runs. You might see this called 'marathon pace', because you can stick to it for a longer time.
3. Tempo or aerobic running
   That step up from easy, which you won't be able to maintain for as long as your steady pace.
4. Threshold or VO$_2$ max
   It's hard now! If you get this pace right, you should find it tough. You're hitting this heart rate during your faster workouts and intervals.
5. Fast–very fast – speedwork/anaerobic/max pace
   It's really tough at the top. You're hitting this heart rate in your hardest running. There's definitely no chat at this pace and you are 'all out' and have that 'heading for the red line' feeling.

Finding out your zones

You can get really scientific with this. If you want to venture into the world of lab testing you can get exact HR zones prescribed to you, but the chances are that you're already accessing some data if you use a GPS or smart watch linked to an app. As a general rule, you can work out your zones by finding out your maximum HR (the hardest you get your heart beating in a hard workout), your resting HR (how slowly it beats at complete rest or when you first wake up) and setting zones between them on scales as outlined above.

Getting to really know the differences between zones that are just for you can help you to get the most from your sessions. You will find a lot of online calculators to help you work these zones out if your wearable GPS watch doesn't do it for you but they may not be completely accurate. Some watches work out your heart rate from the wrist, but we find chest strap monitors are more accurate as wrist monitors can be affected by the fit of your watch, how strong your pulse measurement is at the wrist and even how fast you run, which in turn might set the watch into a different position. If you find you are getting some consistent data back from your wrist, though, it's still valuable and can inform your training in the same way.

The techy bit – heart rate ranges for training

As volume of oxygen consumption increases, so does heart rate (HR). If you want to run at a certain percentage of your maximal oxygen uptake (VO_2) you can estimate it with a simple calculation:

1. First measure your resting HR (RHR) and then measure your maximum HR (MHR).
   E.g. RHR 60, MHR 160
2. Now subtract your resting HR from your maximum HR. This is your HR reserve (HRR).
   E.g. HRR = 160 − 60 = 100
3. If you want to run at 80 per cent of your VO_2 max, simply take 80 per cent of your HR reserve and add your resting HR to that. The sum is your target HR for running at 80 per cent VO_2 max.
   E.g. 80% of 100 = 80 + 60 = 140bpm

Your target HR for 80 per cent VO_2 max is therefore 140bpm.

As we said above, the goal of effective, progressive and well-structured training is that as your training progresses you will be able to run faster at the same or lower heart rates. While good endurance runners may not always have the highest VO_2 max, improving VO_2 max does mean a better 'aerobic ability', allowing faster running for longer. For many years, it was the commonly held belief that that long, slow-distance (LSD) running was the most effective training for increasing VO_2 max, but recent scientific evidence suggests otherwise. Training must be specific to be effective and so LSD is unlikely to improve your high-intensity ability (VO_2 max) the most. The solution to this problem is to reduce training volume and increase training intensity. Reported studies show that training at 80–90 per cent of your VO_2 max (remember this is equivalent to 80–90 per cent of your HR reserve plus resting HR) produces the greatest benefit for improving an athlete's 'aerobic ability'.

Let's take a look at some example HRR ranges, the same as those used above, and some example running sessions for each. There are more session examples later in the chapter.

- Recovery or easy running = less than 59 per cent HRR (great for LSD and active recovery). Session example: 90-minute easy run.
- Steady running = 60–70 per cent HRR (good for base mileage). Session example: 40-minute base run.
- Tempo running = 71–79 per cent HRR (good for running economy). Session example: 2 x 15-minutes at tempo intensity with 5-minute jog recovery between each.
- Threshold running = 80–89 per cent HRR (good for running economy). Session example: 4 x 6-minutes at threshold intensity with 3-minute jog recovery between each.
- Fast running = 90–95 per cent HRR (intervals – good for improving VO_2 max and speed endurance). Session example: 6 x 3-minute efforts, with 4-minute jog recovery between each.
- Very fast running = >95 per cent HRR (speed work – good for improving VO_2 max). Session example: 6 x 200m efforts with 400m jog recovery between each.

KNOW THE LINGO: TRAINING TERMINOLOGY

It really doesn't need to be complicated. We don't want to throw tricky words at you to show our level of understanding (or the gaps in it, depending on how you look at it!) but we do want to help you relate to some of the jargon you'll typically see to help you understand some common training terms and to see how they apply and can fit, or not, in your training ingredients. When you understand what you're doing, and why you're doing it, you can take more ownership of it and it has greater potential impact and training benefit.

Aerobic or anaerobic running

Your body can make energy with oxygen (aerobic) or without oxygen (anaerobic). However, you never make 100 per cent of your energy aerobically or anaerobically, so in that sense pure aerobic or anaerobic running doesn't really exist. But, for purposes here, let's call running that requires most energy to be made anaerobically 'anaerobic running' and running that allows most energy to be most aerobically 'aerobic running'. Energy produced aerobically is more efficient (i.e. more energy per unit of glucose fuel) but takes longer to produce and is therefore useful during lower-intensity exercise when your body's energy requirements are lower. Because of the lower intensity and efficient energy production, aerobic running can be sustained for longer periods of time. On the other hand, lots of energy can be made anaerobically in a short space of time, but this is inefficient (i.e. not much energy per unit of glucose fuel). Because lots of energy can be produced quickly, high-intensity, anaerobic running is possible, but it cannot be sustained for more than a few minutes at a time, although not because you run out of fuel (*see* lactate on p. 112). So, 100m runners predominantly make their energy anaerobically and marathon runners predominantly make their energy aerobically.

If your body is better at producing energy aerobically you will be able to run faster for longer – the goal for most runners. So, we should only run aerobically to improve that system, right? Well, in fact both aerobic and anaerobic running will improve your 'aerobic ability'. An improved 'aerobic ability' means your aerobic energy system can keep up with a higher intensity of running and you are able to sustain this for longer periods of time – essential for successful marathon running.

Endurance runners typically engage in aerobic running to boost their stamina and endurance base. Great aerobic base sessions include long, slow runs, relaxed, low-intensity and in control, where time on feet is the focus. This is especially important for long-distance runners who need to optimise their efficiency. However, runners keen to improve their aerobic ability certainly shouldn't neglect faster- and varied-paced running in their training programmes if they want to really boost aerobic ability.

Running economy

Here, we're talking about fuel economy (*see* Chapter 5 for further information on nutrition). Glucose is the preferred fuel of working muscle, especially as exercise intensity increases. However, glucose is in relatively short supply. You don't have enough stored glucose to run a marathon at any pace. How, then, can runners improve their ability to work really hard for long periods of time? To do that we need better access to a stored fuel source that contains lots of potential energy: fat. Fat contains about twice as much energy as glucose, but it's harder to get at and the process of transforming it into energy requires more oxygen (think 'aerobic ability'). It's important to retain some of your glucose store during running because efficient use of fat as a fuel requires glucose. Several changes occur after aerobic training, including getting better at transporting fat into muscle and an increased efficiency at getting the energy from that fat. Keep this in mind when you're wondering why you're doing threshold runs. They really do help you become more economical, allowing you to run harder for longer, turbo diesel style.

The key for most endurance runners is to become more economical. That is, they become better at using available fuel stores for faster running. Threshold running, or running with 'tolerable' or 'controlled' discomfort, is great for boosting running economy over longer distances.

VO$_2$ max

VO$_2$ max is the giant of key terms used in sports science and it is so often misunderstood. Let's break it down to its 'bare bones' and start with the abbreviation itself: V = volume, O$_2$ = oxygen and max = maximum. It is the maximum volume of oxygen that your body can consume. There are two very important parts to this. First, how good your heart is at pumping oxygen containing blood to working muscles, and second how good your muscles are at extracting oxygen from that blood.

Why do runners need to know this? The greater your capacity to consume oxygen, the longer and harder you can run while still making the most of your energy aerobically. So the best marathon runners will have the highest VO$_2$ max, right? No, not always. In fact, the length of marathons means that athletes do not run at or close to their VO$_2$ max, unlike middle-distance runners, and therefore a very high VO$_2$ max is not as critical. However, successful marathon runners *are* highly efficient at consuming oxygen, giving them a fairly high VO$_2$ max and excellent running economy. Training that improves your VO$_2$ max, such as interval training, high-intensity running, and, to an extent, threshold running, will help your marathon performance, but don't assume you will be a better marathon runner just because your VO$_2$ max is higher than that of the athlete running next to you. Although VO$_2$ max can be increased with training, the effects are not as marked as those that can be realised through effective training designed to train you to run more economically!

Perceived exertion – 'how does it 'feel'?

Perceived exertion (or 'rating of perceived effort', RPE) is a very useful and reliable way to gauge running pace. Runners are becoming increasingly reliant upon external indicators of exercise intensity and tools for measurement, such as wearable GPS trackers. These certainly provide excellent tools for helping understanding, yet to some extent they take away the need for runners to listen, interpret and understand the physical sensations they experience when running at different intensities. For example, we can all imagine running at different intensities will 'feel' different; an easy run feels very different from a threshold run. As your training progresses and you improve, you will be able to run faster and longer with the same 'feel'. Cast aside and leave behind your watch every now and again and learn to use your internal perceptions to guide and judge your effort level. Don't become slaves to modern technology, don't let it set your boundaries or provide limitations, instead, use it to run faster!

Lactate

Rewind for a moment. Lactate is the most frequently misunderstand science-y term! Let's dispel some myths. Lactic acid and lactate *are not the same thing* (one hydrogen ion difference), although lactic acid quickly becomes lactate in your body's cells. So, when talking about lactic acid you are basically talking about lactate since the former rapidly becomes the latter. Also, lactate is *not* a waste product, a toxin to be massaged out of muscle or the cause of delayed onset muscle soreness (DOMS – *see* p. 113). In fact, lactate is essential for energy production and is a preferred fuel for many organs, including the brain and heart. So, lactate is our friend and not necessarily a foe.

However, you can have too much of a good thing! High-intensity, anaerobic running will produce more lactate than can be used or removed and so it begins to accumulate in muscle and blood. At a certain running intensity, lactate accumulates in your blood rapidly and is associated with a percentage of your VO_2 max. We can call this intensity or percentage VO_2 max either 'lactate threshold' or 'onset of blood lactate accumulation'. Theoretically, accumulating lactate, during anaerobic running, is associated with premature muscle fatigue and suppressed energy production; neither of which are effective for running.

Through specific running training you can increase the running intensity and percentage of your VO_2 max at which you can run before blood lactate accumulates, improving your ability to run at a harder pace for long periods of time. Here is where the term 'threshold' running really comes into its own and why running under controlled discomfort is a good descriptor of this pace. Effective threshold-paced running sees you control a pace that is bang on, or just under, the point at which lactate accumulates faster than it can be removed or used. The right balance of the right training sees the speed of this pace increase over time.

Delayed onset muscle soreness (DOMS)

The muscle soreness you get 24–48 hours after hard training is not a build-up of lactate or any other toxin. In fact, lactate only hangs around in your body, as lactate, for about 15 minutes after exercise. Think about it, do you always get sore muscles? No. Do you always produce lactate during training? Yes.

The cause of DOMS (remember Tuesday legs?) is not entirely clear, but what is known is that exercising in an unaccustomed manner causes tiny injuries to muscles. The presence of the injury causes inflammation and swelling. The inflammatory fluid contains substances that cause further muscle breakdown, leading to pain. The muscle is repaired and the discomfort subsides. The bad news is that there is not much you can do about DOMS. A thorough warm-up before your training session may reduce the severity to which you experience DOMS because the warm-up will decrease the extent to which you are unaccustomed to the training you are about to perform. Remember, the length of your warm-up should increase if you plan to train at a high intensity and the warm-up should be specific to the training session. In general, a proper warm-up should last between 5 and 20 minutes, depending on how hard you plan to run. If you suffer from severe DOMS frequently then perhaps your training programme progression is too aggressive. Equally, DOMS is difficult to avoid, since training load for improvement should be progressive and therefore you should be frequently exposing yourself to exercise that you are not accustomed to in order to reap the benefits of training!

A PHASED APPROACH TO PLANNING

Ever pitched up to a race and thought to yourself: 'I've nailed my build-up for this race, my planning was brilliant. I'm as ready as I can be right now?' That's the ideal physical and mental state with which to hit race day. Ready to rock. Ready to execute. Such confidence comes from great training and great training comes from great planning. OK, so there's a caveat here: it doesn't need to be perfect! We don't believe in the old 'be the best you can be, no pain no gain, perfect practice makes for perfection' approach. We know it isn't going to always go to plan, but experience tells us that developing an overall framework for your planning that moves you through well thought-out cycles and phases not only keeps your training fresh, variable and targeted, but also keeps you motivated, on track and progressing. It also puts you in the best possible place to be able to plan your approach properly and realise the types of outcomes that will make you smile.

When you break your approach to training up into manageable cycles it gives focus and clarity for each phase. This is known a 'periodised' approach and in endurance running that means knowing what running to do when and in what amounts in such a way that fits your challenge, your context and your commitment. This means breaking training up into smaller focused chunks and phases, each with a distinct and sometimes different focus. You can't expect to jump from your base level of fitness to your best race performance in one or two weeks. It's a much more enjoyable and rewarding process – and we are all about process – to build gradually to peak fitness. What's more, you're less likely to burn out when it's done with a patient, measured and planned build-up. The phases outlined below work well for endurance runners.

Start with the date of your A race and work backwards building in the phases to take you from preparation to perfection.

Aerobic conditioning/base/preparation phase

Allow four to six weeks. This phase is about constructing an aerobic base and establishing a robust training profile. Typically, running during this phase is low in intensity and focuses on building the foundations for the training to come. Think of it like building a house. You wouldn't try to put the wiring or plumbing in before the footings, walls and roof were in place. A strong, robust and healthy foundation allows you to layer subsequent training on top. This phase improves the capacity of the heart, lungs and muscles to use oxygen more effectively and deliver it to the working muscles. It also helps muscles, bones and tendons grow strong and helps the body to learn to store and utilise fuel for endurance exercise. It's also a good time to establish and integrate your training budget and your training routines and make any changes you need to.

Aerobic conditioning adaptation phase

Allow four to six weeks. This phase progresses the aerobic foundations and begins to bring in some specific conditioning elements. It continues to work on developing the efficiency and economy of your running and builds muscular endurance. It's all about starting to ask tougher questions of yourself and the running you do. Your previous base of steady and easy running will have put you in a strong position – that is, stable, robust and injury-free to tolerate increased workloads and running speeds. The transition from one phase to the next shouldn't be aggressive or sudden but should flow seamlessly, almost as if you don't notice the subtle shifts in emphasis.

Pre-competition adaptation phase

Allow four weeks. This phase really introduces focused specificity to your plan. It's all about building on the successes of the previous two phases and introducing longer, harder workouts and working further on developing your maximal oxygen uptake and running economy. You should be noticing changes to your running speed, heart rate and perceived effort during this phase. Running faster for longer should be becoming easier!

Sharpening/competition phase

Allow four weeks. This phase involves you putting the icing on the cake as your A race draws closer. It adds the final touches to your grand scheme. It's often in this phase that runners start to doubt the training that has taken place before and cram too much of the wrong types of training in too close to their big race. Be confident at this time and trust the training that you have done. As your A race draws near, volume drops significantly and a taper period allows your body to reach peak performance. We will get more into what tapering looks like in Chapter 6.

THE ELEMENTS OF A PERFECT TRAINING PLAN

Remember, any training plan should fit into your life. It's a mistake to try to squeeze or wrestle a training plan (especially an optimistic one) into your life. Making you fit the plan won't work. Make the plan fit you.

Reflect again on your goals and training budget before you start to put it together! Don't try to write your whole year or long cycle in one go. Chop it up using the periodisation/phases we got into above. Then think macro, meso and micro cycles:

- A macro cycle is often a year or more if you're building towards a big or long race event. Macro cycles to you might look like a race calendar filled with familiar races in seasons, such as always working towards cross country in the winter, or a track race in the summer. Everyone's macro cycle will look different depending on aspirations.

- Meso cycles are that bit in between that you probably spend most of your time looking at – the 'training plan' you download, write on, personalise, stick on your fridge, programme into your phone.

- Micro cycles are the chopping of that further into weekly plans focused on the workouts, runs and rest days you do day by day. Your micro cycles definitely should be the most discussed, flexible and process-driven parts of your training, and should include the following components outlined below.

Dates

A good training plan should be dated and planned towards your goal race or event. While days, weeks and dates are important to keep you on track, they don't need to be so rigid that you become a prisoner to them. Allow flexibility for your lifestyle and any niggles or illness you might encounter. Give yourself freedom. Play with it. Personalise it.

Easy runs

Easy runs form your aerobic base and they are vital for recovery from hard sessions. Some coaches advise that as much as 80 per cent of your week should be at easy pace, but this will depend on your goal and the time you have to run each week. Easy runs should be conversational pace, comfortable and enjoyable. Make sure you're dialled into a pace that feels a little 'too' slow and keep your heart rate low.

Workouts

There should be at least one hard workout a week, whatever you're working towards. What this looks like will depend on what you're training for and your personal aspirations. Some training plans will have more than this but it will depend on the training budget you have (time to spend) and how you respond to the quality of the workout in terms of recovery, whether you need or indeed should have any more. Doing one workout or 'session' once a week that makes you feel like you're running out of your skin is a great start.

Rest

Planned rest days are the best days! Plan your rest days where they give you the best chance to recover from a session, prepare you for a longer run or race and fit best around work. How many rest days you need per week depends on what you're training for, the miles you're putting in, and how you cope with an increase in miles and/or workload. Make sure you have at least one planned rest day per week and experiment with moving this around. Rest days are when your body responds to the training you've been doing so remember this if you're struggling to stop!

Strength

Not just 'lifting weights'. Include something strength based, whatever that looks like for you. You might go to the gym, do bodyweight or resistance band exercises, a Pilates class or a set routine from a strength coach or physio. Again, it's great to plan this in your training at least once a week. Let it stand alone as a workout rather than being tagged on after a run – you'll be more likely to do it properly and get more from it. Remind yourself of some of the basic ideas for strength exercises given in Chapter 3.

Build-up races and benchmarks

It's a good idea to include these to allow yourself opportunities to practise pacing, kit and nutrition. It's different nailing your pacing alone compared to in a racing environment and races will help you to grow in confidence in your build-up. You don't have to go all out and do this regularly, but make sure you have at least one planned. We are huge fans of using our parkruns for this, whether that's as a regular test of fitness by running at goal pace, or popping a parkrun in the middle of a longer workout: aka 'the parkrun sandwich'.

Golden rules for planning

- Be realistic but challenging, be progressive yet stable, and be consistent.
- Tailor your programme to fit with your lifestyle and don't expect things to flow seamlessly without a blip!
- Be responsive. Following your plan religiously isn't compulsory! It is far better to allow for pressure points, whether they are work, domestic or social related, and work round them with your training rather than have them cause a total stop.
- Maintain a balance of recovery – stress – progression. Most training adaptation will come when you are resting, so remember that. Easy running is a key ingredient throughout. Hard – easy – hard works.
- Learn to listen to your body. More isn't necessarily better. If you're tired, rest.

- Be prepared to accept where you are in your phase of training and acknowledge that you won't (and arguably shouldn't) try to be at peak fitness all the time. Give yourself room to improve and be patient.

- Endurance training benefits take time to develop. There are no magic potions or quick fixes. Be patient and give your body time to adapt to the appropriate application of workload and recovery.

GET TO GRIPS WITH WORKOUTS

When considering your route to movement in the midpack, all the fundamentals of training, the pillars, the principles of training, the basics of different types of running and the rules of planning matter, but the day-to-day ingredients of your core workouts, the money miles, the workouts that help you strive towards your goals, are vital. The way in which these are planned, scheduled, prepared for and executed really matters in the grand scheme of progressing your running, nourishing your running and finding joy in your running. If you want to move in the midpack, you've simply got to plan and run the workouts that matter, that are relevant to your running aspirations and that will make the difference on race day.

We are going to share a few workout ideas over the next few pages. These by no means constitute an exhaustive catalogue of training sessions, just a guide to help you develop a few different ideas and navigate your way in training towards better running, whatever that means for you.

We've outlined these workouts based on aspirational race distances of going faster (5km/3.1 miles), getting stronger (10km/6.2 miles), going the distance (half marathon) and going longer (marathon).

SO YOU WANT TO GO FASTER (5K AND UNDER)?

Faster workouts are great to add in to any training programme to increase your fitness, even if your long-term goal is to run something longer. Real speed is something you might neglect in favour of staying cosy in your comfy aerobic blanket. Even if your racing goals are aimed at running 10km (6.2 miles) and more, keeping on top of your speed work will almost certainly improve your performance. Fast running develops neuromuscular conditioning, boosts your VO_2 max, improves your tolerance for lactate build-up (thus training a different energy system), improves running economy and helps promote better technique and form. It develops that 'kick' that you feel as the gears shift when you're heading to a finish line. In short, it's ace. Speed training will definitely get you out of breath, your heart pounding and muscles screaming. That's the point.

If you're working towards a mile or trying to improve your parkrun time, we suggest doing a few faster runs per week if your training budget allows, and once a week for everyone else. It doesn't have to be done on a track (although of course there are benefits to doing them there – no traffic disruption, good surface, flat) but you should choose somewhere that's good underfoot with a good safe surface on which you can run flat out. Again, the way you do your speed sessions is a personal thing. Some runners will get the best out of themselves doing them alone with music pumping through earphones, while others will need the pull-along of running in a group and injecting competition. Work out, too, when is a good time of day to do fast workouts like these. Some run faster in the mornings, others later in the day. It's a good idea to also stick a few workouts in around the time you will be doing your goal race. If you've only ever run fast in the evening, it's hard to get your body to shift into that gear if it's a morning race unless you've prepared for it.

Midpack workouts

1. Back-to-backs

These are 100m fast runs with very short recoveries. For instance, 12 x 100m sprints with 15–30-second jogged turnarounds. Even for the fittest out there this simple speed session is tough if done correctly. Each 100m should focus on form, stride length, quick cadence, strong drive and quick acceleration to top speed. After each run, don't come to an abrupt stop. Slow down, turn around and repeat. Hold on to form all the way through, including for the tough final 4 x 100m runs.

2. Coe 300s

Olympic 1500m champ in 1980 and 1984, Seb Coe completed this flat-out session as his acid test of readiness for major championships. He'd cover each 300m in 35–38 seconds (that's 52-second 400m pace!), but we don't expect you to be quite that swift.

Run 6 x 300m with 2:1 recovery – i.e. if each 300m takes 60 seconds, take a 2-minute walk/jog recovery. Remember, run them hard!

3. Down the clock

Increase your running speed with the decrease in distance – 500m – 400m – 300m – 200m – 100m – (double the time it took you to run each rep as recovery).

Once this session has been mastered in terms of running faster for each distance, the session can be progressed: 1) add a second set; 2) reduce the length of recovery between efforts. Play with this session and monitor how you progress.

4. Flat out 4s

This is a classic session performed over 400m. It consists of 8 x 400m, each one run at target mile time with 4–6 minutes' jogging recovery between each interval. In this session, the focus is on 'best pace' for each 400m and across all 400m efforts. It's not about running the first and last effort as flat-out efforts with the ones in the middle being seconds slower. Run consistently and go for a repeatable 'hard best pace'.

5. Jelly legs

This session is about completing a maximal effort, recovering and then trying to maintain that same pace over shorter distances. Run 3 minutes flat out (60 seconds' recovery), then run 6 x 30 seconds flat out (2 minutes' recovery between each one).

To progress this workout, repeat the set a second time after a full recovery.

6. The Yelling classic

This is a firm favourite of ours and a great test of fitness at the start and end of a training cycle. Run 6 sets of 3-minute intervals hard with

90 seconds' jog recovery between each. Aim for controlled, hard running that is consistent. Look back on this workout when you repeat it and see the progress you've made.

SO YOU WANT TO GET STRONGER (10K)?

Mastering control of your pace is important when you're working towards a 10km (6.2-mile) race. For a great 10k and beyond, you should be teaching your body to tolerate anticipated race day pace, intensity and duration. This is the same whether your race is on the roads or trail. You need to build a strong aerobic base with great endurance, and that needs to happen over time, so look back on the guidance on periodisation and get ready to get stuck into the long game.

Great 10k training should be predominantly aerobic (steady runs, threshold runs and longer intervals) but it pays to include regular top-end speed sessions, as outlined in the 'So you want to go faster?' section on p. 119. Using the different energy systems regularly in your training means your body is going to be ready to face whatever you throw at it come race day. We like doing 10k workouts on the road where we can. Roads with a good surface and some undulation will make you stronger and ready to tolerate anything a race might have in store for you, but remember to do some workouts on the terrain you've chosen to race over, too. Make it as specific as you can for good results, and don't forget to add warm-up, cool-down and stretching time.

Midpack workouts

1. Mile reps

Mile repeats are classic 10k training territory. On an accurate, measured mile (1.6km), run 5 x 1-mile repeats at your target 10k race pace. Take 2 minutes' recovery between each mile repeat. Running intervals at a pace that is at (or very close to) your 10k race pace helps you learn to tolerate your desired pace and adapt to this intensity. Be careful not to go off too hard for the first few reps!

2. Killer hills

On a hill that takes you 90 seconds to run hard from bottom to top, complete: 6 x 90-second runs; 6 x 60-second runs; and 6 x 30-second runs. Each hill effort should be as fast you can manage and best pace for the full session. At the top of each interval, turn around and jog back down the hill as recovery. Hill running builds leg strength and stamina, which is important for great 10k control. Running a strong set of hill repeats demands a tough mindset and is a great way to tick off mileage without having to go too far.

3. The chipper

You're going to run 12-, 10- and 8-minute segments starting at your tempo effort and getting faster each time. Take 3-minute jog recoveries between each interval to get yourself feeling fresh again. By the last section, you should be pushing into threshold but in the cruise zone, keeping everything controlled as you smash it out.

SO YOU WANT TO GO FOR DISTANCE (HALF MARATHON)?

A half marathon really is a great racing distance. It's far enough to stretch you but without the extra training demands (time from your training budget, especially) of a full marathon. A half marathon is a perfect way to stretch a few boundaries, run further or faster than before, and can be a very realistic and achievable goal for you to work towards. Good half marathon times can sometimes happen when you're training for something longer because you've built an engine that has good aerobic base and can tolerate long durations. Great half marathons have heaps of controlled steady and easy running in the build-up with time spent on longer pace-controlled running into threshold. To complete your best half marathon you need speed, endurance and the ability to keep focused and on the pace when the going gets tough. Winding up the pace and picking it up further into a run will help you develop your aerobic capacity and your ability to keep your pace on track in the latter stages of your race.

Midpack workouts

1. The pick-up

Run 20 minutes at a steady pace 'out' in one direction. This pace should be in the region of 20–30 seconds/mile (12–18 seconds/km) slower than your target half marathon pace. After 20 minutes, turn around and retrace your steps back over the route you have just run, but at a faster pace. The goal is to complete the 20 minutes on the way back faster (i.e. get further and continue past the start point) than you did on the way out.

2. Chase the threshold

Threshold running is your best friend for a great half, especially into the middle phase of your training. Running a better half marathon means being able to push the boundaries of comfort a little further that you might think is possible and running on the edge of your comfort zone for longer. Remember, threshold is around 80 per cent of your effort. Try a session of 3 x 10 minutes' threshold with 2 minutes' jog recovery each time.

3. The perfect pacer

Aim to do this in the second half of your build-up. Run 2 x 4 miles (6.4km) at your target half marathon race pace with 10 minutes' jog/walk recovery between race-paced efforts. This type of session will show your body what target pace feels like for a longer duration and will help you to build confidence as you work towards your goal. Don't be scared of your target pace – relax into it as much as you can in the first effort and the second one will feel easier.

SO YOU WANT TO GO LONGER (26.2 AND BEYOND)?

Whether you're working up to your first full marathon or you've done a few and want to get faster over the classic distance, the key thing to consider is that in a successful build-up you need to lay down the foundations that keep you training well and being injury-free.

A build-up to a marathon should be long – about 16 weeks is optimum – as you aim to spend longer on your feet, learn how you handle longer endurance and practise fuelling, which will and should be different to how you've approached a half marathon. Building up to a marathon or further should ask questions of your stamina, build some adversity and make your endurance aerobic engine bigger than it's been before. The key is always that it's going to take time. Your main aim for longer distances should be to remain consistent and to gradually (and carefully) bank increasing miles. We recommend one long, increasing-distance run per week that is progressive and allows weeks for 'dip', where you can back off and decrease load.

The key components of a build-up to a marathon are long, base, steady miles; tempo and threshold running; some interval running; and a mixture of long runs that are long and easy, long and a little faster, and long with blocks of changing pace in them.

First, let's get something really clear. Don't be fearful of running longer. If you're really anxious about upping the miles, then it's time to calm down. The marathon is a very long run, in fact it's more likely for many to be a very long run with some walking, and for some a very long walk with some running! Whatever your approach, that's fine, but what won't change is the requirement to run, jog, walk or crawl 26.2 miles (42.2km). Instead of being anxious about upping the distance of your longest runs over the next couple of months, embrace the benefits that go hand in hand with going long.

Why are long runs so good for you?

Long runs build the stamina and endurance that is vital for marathon success. They develop your running efficiency, your cardio and respiratory systems (heart and lungs) and the strength and sustainability of your muscles, bones and joints. In addition, and importantly, they teach you how to keep going when you want to stop. Long runs prepare you both physically and mentally for the demands of a sustained time on your feet and what's to come on race day.

What is a long run?

The distance of a long run varies depending on a person's experience, fitness, marathon aspirations and motivation. For some novice marathoners, a long run may well be in the region of 10 miles (16km). An experienced PB-hunting marathon campaigner may be racking up regular miles in excess of double that. The key to 'long' is what is long *for you* and what *you* need to do to build your physical confidence and competence so you can run 26.2 miles (42.2km). You certainly don't need to run 26.2 miles (42.2km) in training, nor do you need to bang out week after week of painfully long miles. But you do need to look to progress your long runs so you can manage between 18 and 22 miles (29–35km) at around three weeks before race day.

How fast is a long run?

The pace of a long run depends on the fitness, experience, aspirations and motivation of the person running it. The simple rule is that the longer you are running for, the slower you should be running. In order to keep going for longer, and for the pace and effort to be sustainable, it's essential to learn how to be efficient, controlled and economical. A good guide here is your degree of breathlessness. Where your breathing rate is controlled, you can hold a conversation, the pace feels manageable and you can keep going. What feels 'easy' (for example, an effort level of 5 out of 10) at the start of a long run won't stay that way as the duration continues to increase (where the effort required to hold the same pace will inevitably go up). For longer runs, it's the distance not the intensity that causes fatigue. The effort required might go up as the distance covered increases, but the pace will remain constant. At least, that's your goal!

Long runs: what can you expect?

Unlike with trying to run faster, where it's the intensity that causes you to slow down, it's the duration that causes the stress and discomfort when going long. The trick of mastering the long run is to start off at a predetermined effort or pace, keep going and minimise (or remove) the rate of slow-down. Successful distance runners have an ability to tolerate discomfort for an incredibly long time. Blisters, chafing, deep muscle ache, thirst, hunger, depleted energy levels and strength and motivation to keep going are all factors in long run success.

Four ways to own your long runs

1. Progress

What is your longest run to date (e.g. 10 miles/16km) and what is your aspirational long run distance (e.g. 26.2 miles/42.2km)? Add miles gradually and progressively and see your long runs as stepping stones to your overall distance target. Running smart long runs should see your overall strength, stamina, fitness and conditioning improve as the weeks and months progress and not break you down and leave you feeling tired and battered. If that's the case, you've clearly done too much too quickly. Don't rush progress, be patient and steady. The best foundations are laid slowly over a long period of time. Be gentle, consistent, build up appropriately and progressively for you, just a few miles or minutes a week, and stick with it. If you're up to 10 miles (16km), you've got plenty of time to realistically build to 20 miles (32km) over the cycle of your training.

2. Fuel

One thing you'll certainly notice as you start to tick the big miles off is the demand that this places on your energy reserves. When you run slower you are working a different energy system than when running faster. We've all got enough fat supplies to keep going for ages and ages at a very slow speed but very few of us are conditioned well enough to be able to access and effectively utilise those stores. It is possible to teach yourself to be more 'fat oxidative' on longer runs (for example, through fasted long slow runs) but these adaptations take time. Most of us need to think about the ways in which we keep our body as tip-top as we can when going long and consider taking some fluids and fuel with us. To be sensible and safe, when you're running for longer, have some fluids and food accessible. Just what you choose to take on your long runs to fuel and hydrate you will vary from person to person. Your long run in training gives you the perfect opportunity to trial and retrial your energy sources and requirements so you feel ready to put your strategy in place on race day. We are going to get into this in our Chapter 5 on Nutrition.

3. Pace

Pacing your marathon is perhaps the most important aspect of getting race day right. It's easy to get excited and forget the best-laid plans of starting slowly, and go off too fast. Starting too fast makes running the second half of the race very tough indeed! You need to learn how to control your pace and run an even and well-paced marathon. It's your long runs in training that give you the awareness of pace and distance, the experience of how it feels, the courage to keep going and the confidence to finish.

To begin with, long runs are best done at a controlled and manageable pace – perhaps 45–60 seconds/mile (28–37 seconds/km) slower than your target marathon pace. On a long run, it is the fatigue of the duration that you are training your body to handle. What feels controlled at the start will get harder to maintain as the run progresses. Your target on a long run is to not slow down.

As your stamina improves, it's both relevant and recommended to include some miles at target marathon pace in your long runs. Even if your marathon race goal is to survive and finish, you should know your target pace to within a few seconds/mile. This will give you confidence that you are in control in the early stages of your race and are on track to reach your goals throughout the race. Long runs in training are the perfect learning ground for understanding and perfecting pace control.

Knowing your pace is about understanding what effort you can sustain for the duration of a marathon. It's about having the patience at the start, feeling in control, feeling confident and the master of your race, and being ready to face the demands of the final stages feeling fresher, stronger, more focused and bang on target. You might not be totally sure of this right now, but with long run experience this will become more apparent.

4. Mind

Perhaps the toughest challenge you'll face on your long runs is in your own head (*see* Chapter 2 for a proper dig into this). Before you've even set off you might be talking yourself out of it, convincing yourself that you can't do it, and thinking of reasons not to go. Once you are out there running, that naughty inner you might start harping away that you're not good enough, that the marathon is a step too far for you, that you've bitten off too much this time, that you are so tired you need to slow down, stop, go home. Yep, all normal! One of the wonderful things about running longer in training is that you get to tackle these negative self-sabotaging thoughts, emotions and anxieties head-on and build yourself an armoury of positivity to get through race day. There really is no glossing over the fact that at times your marathon might feel like something you wished you hadn't signed up for. It's going to test your sinews and your synapses. It's going to challenge your own perceptions of your boundaries and you are going to ask physical and mental questions of yourself and visit places in your body and mind you've never been before. That's marathon running. Here's the great news: long runs prepare you for that. Raising your awareness of what's to come helps you develop and select positive psychological strategies that work for you and that you can call on when the demons come knocking, as they inevitably will, in the latter stages of your marathon.

Instead of just churning out your long runs as the same pace week in week out, running long runs differently can really add an extra dimension to your training, especially if you're looking for that marathon PB.

Midpack workouts

1. Long runs more often
Achieve greater marathon success by including more long runs more often. Start your long run build-up earlier and include six or more long runs of 18–22 miles (29–35.4km) in duration. Stringing together blocks of long runs really helps boost your specific marathon endurance. A word of caution, however – remember the importance of balance and recovery when you structure your plan and in particular your long runs.

2. Long runs faster
Pick up the pace of your long run and add a progressive intention. You can try doing this in different ways. For example, try running the entire duration of the long run at a faster pace; or do a 'fast finish' long run during which you pick the pace up throughout the course of the long run so that you finish the final few miles at or faster than target marathon pace.

3. Long runs differently

Think of your long runs as specific training sessions and not just an enjoyable social run. They'll probably be one of the hardest of the week. Run on roads to get your legs accustomed to repeated pounding and the intensity of a hard surface. Run some of your long runs solo. Running without the company of others or music teaches you to focus your mind fully on the task at hand. Use your long runs to dial into your marathon pace and lock on to marathon pace during different sections of your long run. A long run (20 miles/32km) completed with the final 8 miles (13km) at bang-on target marathon pace will give you bags of confidence that training is working and you are close to hitting your marathon goal.

4. The sandwich

Run 30 minutes at easy pace, then 4 x 20 minutes at marathon pace effort with 5 minutes of very easy jogging, followed by 10 easy minutes. This type of sandwich run can be tweaked depending on where you are in your training – just add or decrease time to the reps. If you're going longer than marathon, put more easy running at the start and end to increase the overall duration.

5. Liz Yelling pace switch

After a good warm-up (15–20 minutes) of very easy running, switch your pacing from race pace to 'float'. Complete 1 mile (1.6km) at target race pace then complete 2 miles (3.2km) at 45–60 seconds/mile slower for a set distance or time e.g. repeated for 9, 12, 15, 18 or 21 miles depending on target race distance. This session works best in a late phase of training as it ticks off long miles while keeping your mind focused on the pace.

MONITOR IT

Keeping track of training is important; it not only helps you to record what you've done, but it also helps you see your progress, keep checking in with yourself about it, notice when it's going well (a great confidence booster), and see when it's taking a dip (signalling that you need to back off and take a break). Tracking your progress and race results is rewarding, but monitoring how it's making you feel is just as important. Many of you will have apps, linked to watches, linked to other people. Your race times will be stored somewhere (if you want them to be) and you can probably locate them quickly, but remember that monitoring the *process* is just as important in training.

Whether you're using apps and watches or pen and paper journaling (we are a fan of both and they can be done in tandem) it's a good thing to keep an eye on which workouts you find challenging, any that you feel you could do differently, as well as paces and totals, to make sure you're not doing too much or cutting anything out that you should be doing; that's anything from resting to strength days. For women, noting when difficult days come in a cycle can be useful for getting the most out of your running – it can just be as simple as noticing when a run feels harder in a particular week or day of your cycle, and giving it a go at a different stage and seeing if it's easier.

Keeping track of the paces you're able to hit in different sessions and workouts with effort perception is also really useful, and again it's something we advise you keep notes on. Be specific and honest in the feedback you give to yourself – it's totally OK if that easy run doesn't feel easy some days. Monitoring your training in this way helps to inform any changes you need to make, whether that's increasing or decreasing the frequency of harder sessions or making tweaks to the days on which you take rest days.

You're going to hit some bumps in the road. Injury is one of those bumps closely related to progression. Avoiding injury is part of being a regular runner – that goes for everyone. Avoiding injury is about what you do and don't do, and careful avoidance of injury should come mainly through making your training specific and really taking overload carefully as you work towards the end goal. There's often a knife-edge that's played with by runners in the midpack, and we want you to always be mindful of not pushing that and throwing away the progress made by gaining an injury that is avoidable.

DON'T PRESS THE 'DICKHEAD BUTTON'

With all the best planning and greatest intentions, some of your training is going to come down to one very basic decision: are you going to press the 'dickhead button' today? Making sensible and healthy choices keeps your hand away from the button, but there are going to be times when you are challenged by your training that might lead you to being a dickhead and making poor choices. The dickhead button is a danger to you if you are overtraining, not recovering adequately between your workouts, and it's definitely there (flashing bright red) if you decide to keep running with an injury that isn't getting better. You know deep down when you're being a dickhead, because you will have doubts about whether you're doing the right thing.

The rule is simple: 'if in doubt, don't'. If you think a run is too close to pushing you over the edge, don't ignore it, it's not about bravado and ego. You're simply not being clever, sensible or making progress by toughing it out. This is especially important if anything hurts, if you feel really tired, or if your run that day is going to cause any relational aggro! Know when to say no. That run will still be there ripe for the taking another day.

It's way too easy as a midpack runner to get tied up in a training plan and ignore the things that mean you've just pressed the dickhead button. The pressure of a goal race on the calendar means you feel you have to push on through pain or run when you are ill, injured or feeling knackered. Surprise!

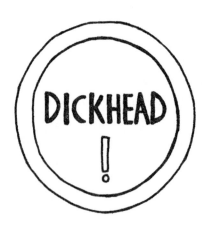

You are making things worse. There are of course things you can run through and you might just feel better by doing so, but as a rule of thumb, you know deep down if you are making it worse. That's when you need to trust the process and know that a few missed days, or weeks, is much better in the long term than something that may cost you a year. We get why it happens (*see* Chapter 2!), but not listening intentionally enough to the signals your body is giving you, inconsistent running and injuries are the biggest potential setbacks to your midpack progress.

As Paul Hobrough says: 'In the last 20 years working with runners of all abilities, one truth comes shining through: runners make choices that aren't always in their best interests.'

Dickhead rules

Be a dickhead
Be a slave to a training plan, neglect good nutrition, neglect relationships, ignore a long-term niggle, burn the candle at both ends, run feeling exhausted, constantly compare yourself to others.

Don't be a dickhead
Get the advice of a professional, keep checking in on your foundations, defer your race place officially, prioritise rest, pull out of the event if you haven't adequately trained for it, do your rehab exercises, show yourself some kindness, exercise patience.

A BETTER RUNNER

Throughout this chapter we've not tried to introduce you to many things that, as a midpack runner, you probably don't know something about already. Types of training, planning your training, fundamentals of training, principles of training, structuring a plan, the rules of progression and workouts to try in your training – all of these things are integrated. They simply don't work in isolation. You will only reap the performance benefits of training if you incorporate it in the right quantities, at the right times, in the right places, aimed at your personal aspirations, with ongoing, sustainable and dedicated commitment.

Training will frustrate you, training will amaze you, training will excite you, training will surprise you. We don't have all the answers to your training. We don't have the scope in this book to address everything you might have on your mind about training. But we do want to encourage you to be curious, to question things you read, to explore training methods, philosophies and approaches (we purposefully haven't spent time debating approaches to these in relation to endurance in this book), but we do want you to understand the basics of how your training impacts upon what you will realise from your running. What you desire from your running is heavily impacted by your approach to training, your experience of training, your training age and wisdom, how you represent your day-to-day, week-by-week and year-on-year approach to training. Training is a very personal thing. Getting it right for you is as much a creative art as it is a science of application. Knowing how to fit the right pieces together at the right times for you is as much about your approach to learning, your mindset, your comfort in change, your ability to flex, adapt, fall and grow as it is about the functional application of simply doing the miles.

The art and science of training is what brings progress to your running achievements. When you get training right, you'll know about it. When it goes wrong, you'll feel that, too. Cultivate progress in your running through understanding why you train, through devoting time to the application of that understanding and knowledge and putting that into what training you do. Most of all, we believe that you will richly nourish your running through executing training that is consistent, enjoyable, progressive, suitable and owned by you. It is when your experience of training is a deeply positive one that you will, without doubt, experience the most joy in your running.

FIVE

NUTRITION

GETTING IT RIGHT

Eating is healthy, normal and something to be enjoyed. In this chapter, we want to present eating as something essential that positively goes hand in hand with running in the midpack. Eating needn't be complicated, it should be simple, yet we know it often isn't. Human beings need food and fluid to survive. Without both we die. Fact. Yet, at the same time, there are many confusing mixed messages, not only with regards to day-to-day healthy eating, but also sports- and running-specific fuelling and hydration, all of which leaves us struggling to filter out what advice is accurate, appropriate or right for us. One thing we do believe is that it takes time and personal investment to truly understand individual everyday healthy eating behaviours and preferences and yet more time and effort to refine these to be effective approaches to eating for running health. You know what does, and doesn't, work for you personally, but sometimes you'll need help realising, discovering, changing and shifting 'what works', and in some cases this will be uncomfortable. Leading sports dietician Renee McGregor reminds us that: 'It is well documented that nutrition plays an integral part in running performance from fuelling and recovery to bone health, mood and motivation and consistency in training. Nutrition, while not rocket science, is also fairly complex.' To be really clear, our focus here is not on 'performance eating' – we believe the whole-body physical and emotional health of a runner is the mainstay of moving through the midpack.

In this chapter, we are going to explain why nutrition is a vital part of moving through and enjoying life in the midpack, and show why nutrition can at times be a very tricky part of the midpack progress puzzle. We are going to explore nutrition as part of the process of being a better runner and a healthier human. We are going to guide you through getting your nutrition right on a day-to-day basis, for training, and for that all-important race day. We are going to get serious about disordered eating in running and what that looks like in the midpack. We know for some runners in the midpack, nutrition can get a little unhealthy. We know some of you are still using your running in some kind of credit/debit system, some of you aren't eating well, others aren't eating enough of what your body needs. We're going to tackle some of that and get you thinking in a much more ordered, healthy and purposeful way. We are definitely going to challenge your thinking, and it may be a little uncomfortable for some of you, but it will be worthwhile.

NO MAGIC RECIPE

Contrary to what you might have been told, read or watched there is no magic recipe for great nutrition for running. We get asked a lot what the best strategy is, especially for racing. We've been asked everything from what's

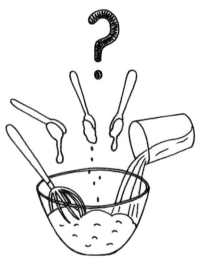

No magic recipe!

the best gel to take on and what's a good recovery drink, to what will prevent me from getting the runner's trots*. Everyone wants to know what's going to give them that extra something, anything, to lift them, especially in the last section of their race. Should they go vegan, go low carb, go no carb, go paleo, go fruitarian, or even run eating baby food (yes, a real question!) or race with beetroot. Everyone seems to be seeking some kind of shortcut magic bean that will lift them out of fatigue and give them some nutritional glory in the last lap/mile/day of their race. Once again, it's test, trial and retrial and personal preference that really matters, although, as we describe later, there are a few clear general healthy guidelines to follow.

Just as many people ask if what they are eating day to day is 'OK', some runners overfocus on using running (and/or exercise) as a reward. You should enjoy exercise and running and you should enjoy food and drink. More of the former doesn't equate to more of the latter, and you especially shouldn't be using terms such as 'allowing yourself X because you ran X miles'. Everyone wants to know if it's OK that they like a beer, and if it's somehow going to damage their running. We've seen some strange habits in running and racing and we're going to do our best to bust some myths and answer some questions.

*Runner's trots: The deadly race destroyer that comes seemingly out of nowhere in the form of desperate, frequent need to visit the toilet. Think lactic legs but deep in your belly. It's often a result of eating or drinking something that doesn't agree with you, or which you have not sufficiently practised consuming. You'll definitely know if you've had this. More on this later.

Nutrition can seem a bit of a minefield

One of the major things we're up against in the midpack – aside from not having a personal chef and nutritionist to look after our day-to-day diet – is that when you start to ask questions it can look like there are nutrition experts everywhere! Just whom can we trust?

We want to enjoy our running, train well and perform when it matters, and we just want to put the right stuff in our bodies to be able to function healthily first and foremost, developing optimal healthy everyday nutrition and a positive relationship with food that underpins and forms the basis of our long, healthy lives and a fulfilling running career.

We are exposed to books, podcasts and online 'experts' with their own unique blend of recommendations and guidance to help us 'eat to run faster'. The major difficulty we have is that to most of us, it all comes across as a lot of ever-changing and conflicting 'wobbly' guidance that isn't backed up with research that's evidence-based. An element of caution is required when wading through quick-fix nutrition guidance to run faster. If it seems there must be a catch, there usually is, even if you can't see it initially.

There's often some online article or study popping up that basically suggests a different approach with every click. This is the kind of overwhelming and unhelpful information overload that makes us switch off and go back to what we were doing in the first place. What's more, being surrounded by runners that are just like us can also lead us to copying what they are doing, even if they are winging it just as much as we are. Very little of what is shouted at us online is science, and none of it is anywhere as unique as you are. Most midpack runners ask coaches like us very basic nutrition questions: 'How do I fuel for X run/workout?'; 'What should I be eating for good recovery?'; 'How do I fuel a great race?'. Get the basics right for you through personal trial, error, test and retest. Learn how your body responds to your daily nutritional choices, good or 'bad'. Reflect on how foods make you feel, train and perform, and use this evidence, and a solid knowledge of the basic fundamentals and good practice in healthy eating in such a way to shape your personal nutrition so that it keeps every bit of your body and mind healthy, responsive and happy.

Sports nutrition is a growing consumer market that can sometimes be confusing to navigate, inconsistent in claims and based on flaky research. Runners can be marketed to easily (if they let it) by companies that target things runners want to improve, as to get better runners will give (almost) anything a try in pursuit of forward movement in the midpack. Sports (running) nutrition is there for us in abundance in gels, shakes, drinks, flapjacks, coffee types, balls, gums and even tablets. They range in price, in promises and in how we can purchase them, whether that's online, in specialist running shops, in supermarkets and at running trade shows. Learning what, if any, sports specific nutrition is best for us is actually part of the process and it's exciting knowing we might not yet have unlocked the thing in nutrition that will play a part in us getting better and creating more joy in our running.

WHAT WE REALLY NEED AND WHY ONE SIZE DOES NOT FIT ALL

We want to start this section by reminding you that we are not qualified dieticians. There are plenty of highly qualified, registered dieticians and doctors with letters after their names who know more about this than we do. However, we've been around the nutrition block a few times, made a few errors, learned a lot, seen heaps of nutrition dilemmas, and helped many runners use their nutrition positively and more effectively to be prepared to train and race. It's not all been glory and optimism, either. Anji has calorie restricted, underfuelled, bonked (completely run out of energy, *see* p. 157), thrown up on the move after overeating before races and definitely taken an unhealthy attitude to 'using' running as a way of earning food. Anji's experiences with nutrition impacted on performance, recovery and injury, especially in the first few years of being a midpack runner, and have made the following years especially difficult. Martin definitely enjoys his food, reaches for the sweet stuff more often that he should, used to train very hard and think this was an excuse to eat anything (and sometimes everything), but has also worked closely with many athletes to help them improve their running by refocusing their personal approach to food and healthy eating.

We aren't experts on nutrition and some of you will know more about fuelling than we do. This is great because you probably got there by good process, great practice and successful outcomes. What we are going to do now is walk you through the basics of some key areas that will hopefully serve as a good, healthy reminder of great practice in nutrition. We are going to give you some ballpark approaches, but we want you to consider that you're all unique, with a massive range of body types, backgrounds, cultural considerations, personal preferences, individual requirements, and demands on your body that range from medical conditions to the goals you have in running. It's vital, with that in mind, that you recognise these figures don't fit everyone and will need you to do some playing around, practising, and, where you can, get some focused support if you need it. Most of all, do your own research on this, find out, explore, discover, refine, trial and work it through.

We really want you to get a good range of great food in and follow a few general guidelines. Eat the good stuff regularly and adjust accordingly depending on your training. We love author and sports nutritionist Anita Bean's idea of eating a rainbow of foods to include a range of vitamins, essential antioxidants and additions to your diet that are much more fun than just taking a supplement in tablet form. Avoiding processed food and sticking with home-made as much as you can, should signal some great nutrition to support not only your running but also your general health.

Once again, we'd like to wholeheartedly reinforce the positive relationship between exercise and eating. You love to run (or you wouldn't be reading this book); therefore, love your food just as much. A simple and effective place to start is to aim for daily nutrition that's rich in mixed food types, as fresh as you can get it, non-processed, contains ingredients whose names you can pronounce (even better if there isn't any packaging), prepared from scratch, and is eaten with company, at a table, with water.

Let's now examine the various elements and types of food we need to include for a really healthy, balanced diet.

Carbs

Carbohydrate might be the biggest and most talked-about element of nutrition for runners. It's definitely the area we have been asked about the most. Traditionally, we were told to carb up and carb load, then more recently to carb cycle, try zero carbs or low carb our way through training and race day. Does anyone really understand what any of that means? Renee McGregor told us that carbs are: 'crucial for optimum performance and progression' while at the same time we have seen high-profile athletes and people like you in the midpack achieve amazing things on a low-carb diet. We are not here to say you should eat this, or shouldn't eat that, and you definitely need to do this; there are multiple ways to skin your carb cat, so once again this is a question of what is really the best way for you.

It's been demonstrated that carbohydrate is a key source of fuel for the body. We can't side step or ignore the fact that carbohydrate is a great source of fuel for runners because it provides energy for every cell of your body – including muscles. Running allows you to burn carbohydrate and fat usefully but how much you need is going to depend on how fast and how far you're going, as well as your body weight. There's a guide for this in Anita Bean's *The Runner's Cookbook*, with a general starting point that if you're running moderately for an hour, you need 5–7g/kg of your body weight in carbs each day. It's important you adjust that up and down for the type of workout you're going to do. If you're going to try a low-carb fuelling strategy, just make sure you get specialist advice on it and make sure it works for you, and that you're doing it for good reasons.

We see carbohydrate as something we can't ignore in running, and Anji in particular has had some good results from getting carb loading 'right' when preparing for longer or more challenging races. You're going to see in all areas of fuelling for running that it's a personal thing that you need to enjoy getting right for you.

Go and get it: pasta, porridge, potatoes, nuts.

Protein

You can't underestimate the value of protein if you want to repair, recover and progress in the midpack. Protein can't be made by your body, but you have to have it if you're going to repair your muscles and get the best from your training. You see protein packed into everything from cereal bars to special milkshakes, but you can't go wrong with basics such as dairy foods, eggs, meat and poultry, and non-animal sources such as soya, nuts and wholegrains. Anita Bean suggests taking on around 0.75g/kg of body weight of protein per day if you're running three times a week, so adjusting this up or down is a very good way to start, depending on how many miles you're putting in. You don't need to smash all your protein in one go after a run or workout, either; Anita suggests spreading your protein intake throughout the day and across your meals, which has the added bonus of leaving you feeling less hungry.

We definitely prefer the approach to protein that suggests we spread it across the day, rather than in one big hit as a powder. It sounds far more enjoyable that we should enjoy nutrient-rich food at every mealtime and this is certainly a method that encourages a healthy approach to eating.

Go and get it: eggs, milk, cheese, chicken, fish, vegetables, nuts, seeds, beans.

Fats

Your body uses fat for fuel, hormone production and to absorb fat-soluble vitamins A, D, E and K into the bloodstream. You can also burn some of it during your running. It's really important to remind you that we're not qualified dieticians, we aren't here to tell you what's 'right' and we certainly don't have the space here to debate, but types of fat and how or when we use them as runners can throw a few different views your way and neither are wrong if they are right for you. The areas you might see some debate in are fat as fuel in running, and fat in everyday nutrition.

Starting with fat in our everyday nutrition, there are two types of fats: saturated fats such as fats found in butter, cakes and biscuits and unsaturated fats like those in avocados, mackerel and seeds. You will come across people advising that some fats should be avoided and others who suggest a low carb (especially white starchy processed carb) and higher fat intake can be beneficial for general health and in some cases even reduce or reverse the risk of diabetes. Professor Tim Noakes is both an author and a scientist in the world of running and an advocate of the LCHF approach as fuel in running and everyday nutrition. There are some organisations like The British Heart Foundation that recommend a low fat approach, suggesting those seeking to lower cholesterol and have general good heart health should seek to focus on consuming less fats.

Secondly, there are differences of opinion and approach with the use of fats to fuel running. There is some debate within endurance running, and especially ultra distance running, in fats versus carbs as fuel for running.

Many agree that some fats aren't great fuel generally (cakes, biscuits etc) for running but there is inconsistency of agreement around the use of unsaturated fats to fuel running. For fat-adapted athletes, particularly those with experience of training in LCHF conditions, their bodies have become more accustomed to accessing and utilising fats as stored fuel. For others, perhaps with more of a carb-based nutritional history, there remains a reliance on carbs for energy.

How you choose to use fat to fuel your running (or not) is an area that should be tried and tested with good intentions, personal practice and always for your own overall health.

Go and get it: salmon, mackerel, avocado, nuts, seeds, milk, cheese.

Fruit and vegetables

These are an easy way to get in a massive range of great vitamins and minerals to support your running through the midpack. It's just an added bonus that they taste great, too. Fruit and vegetables contain high levels of vitamins, and pigments such as beta carotene – great for muscle recovery, oxidants and polyphenols that support your immune system and help you to recover. You'll find vitamin C in citrus fruits as well as red fruits such as strawberries and apples, beta carotene in butternut squash and mango, and vitamin A and C in kale and spinach.

We love smashing a mixture of fruit and veg into smoothies post run, but you can rustle up a perfect post-session dinner by packing them into curries, soups and salads, too.

Go and get it: as wide a range of fruit and veg as possible!

Minerals

There are heaps of minerals that are essential for health, but as this is a running book, we know runner-specific info is what you came for. We've put together a list of our top minerals for runners and where to find them:

- Magnesium – great for strong bones. Find it in leafy greens.
- Zinc – essential in repairing muscle tissue. Get it in red meat and cereals.
- Calcium – vital to avoid low bone density, which is really important for avoiding stress fractures. Mainly in dairy, but if you're vegan find it in leafy greens.
- Vitamin B – useful in producing energy and promoting muscle repair. This can sometimes be missing in female runners, especially around the menopause and after, so go and get it from wholegrains and vegetables.
- Iron – like vitamin B, this can sometimes be low in female runners so bear that in mind because you need it to improve muscle function and capacity. Grab it from red meat and beans.
- Vitamin D – unless you're living and training somewhere with great sunshine, this is likely to be low in your system. You need vitamin D to help you to absorb calcium, which helps your bone density. You'll mainly get it from dairy, but look for foods that have been fortified with vitamin D, such as some types of bread and cereals, too.

Supplements

You will see a whole range of brilliant sources of vitamins and minerals in the lists of foods above, but you might still find there's something missing from your diet that could help you to perform and recover better. Supplements for runners don't just take the form of tablets like a multivitamin, but are available often in gel, bar or drink form, too. We are always going to suggest 'real' food over anything you can pop as a pill, especially where it tastes great and keeps it simple, but if you spot something in the list that you know you're missing, research your supplements before you buy them to make sure they are going to work for you.

Top five nutrition tips

1. Make it personal. This has to work for you and we are all unique.
2. Learn, trial and practise everything.
3. Food is a glorious part of the process. Look for great recipes for nutritious food that gets the best for your training and performance.
4. Avoid processed food as much as you can. Get the good stuff from a balanced and varied diet.
5. The relationship between food and exercise is a great thing. Keep it simple.

SOURCES AND CHOICES

One thing is really clear: not all sources of food are the same. Sure, some foods are cracking sources of carbohydrates – but when that carbohydrate comes from processed, high-sugar, fast-food choices then it simply won't work for healthy, balanced, wholesome, nutrient-rich regular eating. Granted, it'll fill a gap, give you a sugar spike or ping some energy in, but fuel your moving through the midpack for long term? No way José! Food choices and healthy habits embedded every day really make the difference.

If you're really honest with yourself, you know whether your choices are as good as they can be. They usually signal good recovery and have positive effects on how you feel. We are going to look at a couple of debates next that should make you think about sources, choices and why it's great if you make them work for you.

The sugar issue for runners

The challenge of regulating sugar intake is really important for runners to take notice of, without getting overwhelmed by it. Like carbs and zero-carb diets, we see runners following a zero- or low-sugar diet doing just as well as those who include it in their diet. This is something you need to decide for yourself and make your own choices about.

Sugar is an energy source. When you're running, your body uses blood glucose and stored glycogen, which it converts to energy. Most, if not all, energy bars and drinks will contain levels of sugar designed to give you a lift or a hit – we might feel a real genuine sugar buzz after taking them on. It isn't just gels or chocolate bars that can deliver this, either. If you've ever picked up a slice of orange in the later stages of a long race, you will know the hit you can get from natural sugars, too. Unfortunately, the problem with the lift you can get from sugar is the corresponding sugar crash. Some studies on marathon runners have shown that eating a breakfast high in sugar, while guaranteeing a great start with effective glycogen delivery, can bring with it a crash in later stages of the race (*see* our section on bonking on p. 157 for what this might look like). It's about measuring your intake of sugar carefully to make sure you get the benefits of it without suffering for it later in the race.

Making healthy choices when it comes to sugar is really important. We know that if we take on a good breakfast before a race or workout we are going to get better results, as long as it's practised and personalised. Fuelling using some sugar is the same, but we aren't about to suggest you smash a tub of ice cream or stand on the start line eating a bag of sweets. There are good sources of natural sugar, such as bananas, fruit juices and bagels, but again they might contain high levels of sugar that can cause you to spike or crash. It's best to do some research on the amount of sugar you need for your level of activity, in the same way you should with calories, which we are coming to next.

Sugar also gets a bad press because it can be addictive. Cravings for sugar take the form of headaches, tiredness and sometimes stomach pain. And while taking on more sugar than you need can become a bit of an unhealthy cycle, taking too much sugar on in isolation can impact performance, too. Anji heard recently of a midpack runner who was so addicted to fizzy drinks that their running was suffering as they were plagued with stomach problems and regular sugar crashes. Their coach found it really difficult to explain that no amount of training could solve the impact the sugar addiction was having on their running. You need to be able to get the balance right for sugar to work for you as a runner.

Our advice is to research what you need and where possible look for natural sugars. Be mindful of sugar addiction and speak to an expert if you feel it's getting out of hand.

Calories and counting them

Hold tight, here's another nutrition debate! As with the sugar debate, we are going to walk you through some of our thoughts and let you make your own informed choices.

First of all, you have to understand that everyone's requirement for calories is different. Your calorie needs depend on whether you're male or female, your metabolism, your age and how active you are. Even as a regular runner, your requirement will massively change depending on what you're training for. For example, someone regularly running long mileage in training for 50km (31 miles) will have a different requirement to someone who runs 5km (3.1 miles) at easy pace a few times a week. Females will require different amounts at different stages of their cycle. What this means is – you guessed it – this is another area that you need to personalise. Your baseline is to start with 2000 calories for women and 2500 calories for men (current NHS UK guidance) but as with many other areas, you can get a more personalised recommendation if you use a tracking app that takes into account your level of activity and current weight.

The first point we want to make is that not all calories are created equal. It's a stark example, but 'saving up' your calories to have a stack of cakes, crisps and beer at the end of each day isn't going to give you the same goodness from calories spread throughout the day taken from fruit, vegetables and a healthy mix of great home-cooked food. Check out the list of carbs, fats, proteins, minerals and fruit and vegetables above and you'll see a range of foods that contain a varying amount of calories. While we don't want you to deny yourself any food (or groups of them), you will hopefully see where the good nutritional content comes from that will help you to stay healthy as you train, recover and navigate everyday life.

We are often asked about calorie counting as a means of losing weight, especially when people start running as a means of doing so. This is again an area we need you to keep healthy-minded about and we want you to understand the implications of restricting calories as a means of losing weight. Limiting calories has been proposed as a means of weight control and management (and if it is what a dietician or doctor has recommended, do follow their advice), but we would always recommend that you make healthy choices that frame food as fuel to keep you happily and healthily running, rather than as something 'bad' that has to be cut out. Calorie counting, limiting and restricting, in some instances, can be damaging and dangerous if it triggers unhealthy rituals that may lead to injury, underperforming and illness. We are going to talk to you more about unhealthy eating and running in the section on RED-S.

A note on hydration

Hydration is just as important as nutrition and you may have your own strategies for getting that right, especially in longer races. You possibly fall into one of these categories:

- The camel (can store water and rarely feels the need to drink)
- The sipper (little and often)
- The gulper (guzzles water at every opportunity)

Again, your requirements for hydration are a personal thing that you're going to need to practise to get right and won't be the same as anyone else you run with. As you run, you are constantly losing water in sweat, and this is something you need to recognise is happening even during those freezing cold winter runs! The extreme ends of getting hydration wrong are: dehydration, which can affect the pace you're able to maintain and can impact on your health well beyond your training session or race; and hyponatraemia, which essentially floods your body by diluting the sodium levels and can make you seriously ill. In running events, especially those on hot days, it's far more common (and dangerous) for runners to overhydrate and drink too much than to dehydrate. Hyponatraemia is a serious risk for runners. There really is no need to gush down litres of water at every available drinks station. It is important to understand the specific demands of your event, for example extreme conditions, distance, weather and how you respond before, during and after an event. This informs an optimal fluid and hydration strategy for you. Paying attention to your daily fluid intake, your pre-event hydration status and using your thirst as a guide is an appropriate strategy. You can find out your own personal hydration requirements by weighing yourself before and after running, or via a specialist sweat test. These tests might be especially useful if you're running an ultra distance event or in hot or humid conditions.

Hydration can be key in getting your running – especially racing – right and it needs to be considered and practised carefully. Just because you know someone who can go and run two hours straight on a Sunday morning without taking a drink, doesn't mean that's the best strategy for you. Experiment and always ask experts for advice if it's something you feel is impacting on your performance and recovery. You might just unlock a game changer!

Energy drinks

We could write a whole additional chapter on energy drinks and again it's a crowded and slightly confusing market. Energy drinks claim they can improve your performance through sugar, caffeine, isotonics or a mixture of all of these. We can't tell you this enough: whatever you're doing with race nutrition must be practised, and that includes what you're drinking. You might be able to get a great boost from sports drinks, or find they help you in recovery, but don't risk anything new on race day – especially when it comes to caffeine, which may contribute to gastrointestinal (GI) disruption issues (*see* p. 154).

For Anji, energy drinks are a bit of a no-no due to a heart condition and a sensitive stomach, but she does find isotonics useful for recovering from harder workouts since they help to replace salt lost in sweat. Of course, that might not work for everyone. For Martin, it's water and food all the way. We are going to tell you again to personalise it, always read labels carefully, and make sure you are using a drink that is going to work for you.

WHEN A RELATIONSHIP WITH FOOD AND RUNNING ISN'T A HEALTHY ONE

Let's talk about RED-S – otherwise known as 'relative energy deficiency in sport'. It's very real and can be very serious. This certainly isn't something reserved for the super fast elite athletes in tiny shorts. RED-S can affect performance at any level of running, but it can also cause people to become really unwell and lead to complications both physical and psychological that can take years to resolve. It's great that we are now talking more about RED-S and it's important that we are able look for it in ourselves and our running buddies.

RED-S in runners can look like anything from avoiding eating regularly, to binging or starving, to avoiding groups of food completely and anything in between. RED-S can be deliberate in the choices we make, but it can also be the accidental consequence of having a haphazard approach to fuelling for running that is poorly planned and not reactive to training. Symptoms of RED-S present in people as weight loss, lack of energy, frequent injuries, poor sleep and lack of progress in performance, all the way to life-changing things such as poor bone density, skipped and missing periods in women and dangerously low testosterone in men. RED-S doesn't discriminate between fast/slow/short/long distance and it's an issue for men and women in all age groups and in all sports.

We are hearing a lot about midpack athletes presenting at eating disorder clinics with RED-S because they have made unhealthy choices based on aesthetics and a 'lighter is faster' principle. Some runners equate 'you're looking lean' as a compliment that means we look fit and fast, and it gives us a boost. We see all too often runners seemingly performing a balancing act where it's running that holds their eating together, and as soon as injuries happen or other things get in the way, unhealthy eating habits easily slip back.

The first step to opening up about RED-S is starting a dialogue and asking questions of yourself or someone you might be worried about, and that's what we are hoping to prompt in this chapter. Often, thinking about this can get tricky, but nevertheless we are encouraging you to start challenging yourself about these issues. Renee McGregor shared a few stories of runners that might make you think of yourself or someone you run with. Renee has treated those presenting with RED-S at her clinics and shared with us a case study of a university student who had become completely preoccupied with maintaining what he felt was a light enough number on the scales to perform. This runner was fuelling less and training more, notably skipping carbohydrates, and eventually presented at the clinic with extreme fatigue and an increase of injuries. The tests taken undertaken showed extremely high inflammatory markers, extremely low testosterone and a shutting down in his metabolism. Renee explained that not only did he need to take steps to change his eating habits and reset his training, but he also needed a long period of recovery time to get his body back to being healthy enough to perform again.

Just as RED-S isn't reserved for elite runners, neither is the help and support you can receive if you're going through some struggles with your eating. Reaching out to the many organisations out there to help you, such as Train Brave (trainbrave.org), is an important start that will make you a healthier, happier and stronger midpack runner in the long term.

RACE DAY NUTRITION MATTERS

We're going to get into what great racing strategy looks like in Chapter 6, but nutrition is going to play a big part in you getting race day right. We like to think of a car with either no fuel or the wrong fuel in it. Either way, it's not going to get very far before it breaks down, and it's exactly the same for your body.

Race nutrition is important because it can make the difference between a great performance, a finish and a massive bonk, which in running isn't as fun as you'd think. Optimal race day nutrition starts the week before and the day before race day. Get your lead-in fuelling wrong and it'll be too late to do anything about it come race day. Martin experienced this in 2011, prior to running the Comrades Ultra Marathon in South Africa, and before he knew about his wheat intolerance, when he loaded up with pasta the day before the race. Frustratingly, he also 'unloaded' many times in the first 10 miles (16km) of the event as a result, which had a significant impact on energy levels in the later stages of the race. Knowing personal preferences and nutritional responses and practising these so they work ahead of race day is so important.

Race day fuelling begins the day before the race, and continues on the day starting with breakfast. By the time you get to your target race you should have a pretty good handle on what works for you. If you're staying away from home for your race, plan to have something as close to the same as what you'd have at home, and if you're at home make sure you've got whatever it is in stock. Don't add to any pre-race stress the night before by making a last-minute dash to the shops for your breakfast. Part of the training process should be learning what you can stomach before you run, and at what time. Timing is everything because it will signal to your body the timetable counting down to the start of your race – and that includes what time(s) you will visit the loo. Good toilet trip planning reduces the risk of runner's trots and definitely needs to be considered to be of great importance.

Understand the nutritional demands of your event

What you need to fuel your race will vary massively depending on the distance and intensity you're going to run and your personal aspirations. You know by now that what you need to eat and drink before a weekly trot around parkrun isn't the same as what you'll need for a half marathon, and neither is this the same for a marathon or multi-day ultra. The general rule is that you can run for around 90 minutes on stored fuel, but again this will depend on what you've stored and how much effort you're putting into your race. After that, you need to consider fuelling as you go. This is something that's vital to practise in the weeks leading up to your race because you're going to very quickly find out what works for you and gives you the best delivery of energy. We are big fans of fuelling with 'real' food wherever you can, as well as with the traditional gels and performance food on offer. It tends to be the ultra runners among us who have the great ideas for 'real' fuel (and how to carry them), such as sandwiches, snacks and, in one anecdote, someone who learned to run at pace while eating a pot of instant porridge. Maybe this is part of the allure of super-long distance? Find out the general guidance about eating frequency for the fuel you're using and, again, practise this in training.

Just because someone suggests you should take it on every 45 minutes doesn't mean your gut will agree with that.

Race nutrition both before the event and on the day is a highly personal thing that shouldn't be something you're ever tempted to just guess on the day. We've seen some quirky approaches to race fuelling over the years, with everything from someone strapping 10 gel packets to their arm with gaffer tape to someone with bacon taped to the crossbar of their bike in a triathlon. The point is that for them, it obviously worked. You don't get to the bacon idea on guess work alone...

What's often overlooked when it comes to the execution of great race nutrition is practising it at pace. It's one thing getting your on-the-go race fuel open and consumed during an easy run when you're able to stop if you need to, but it's quite another doing it at your race pace. The same goes for carrying it, too. Make sure in your last couple of runs before your race that you are practising carrying and eating at pace as part of a really important final dress rehearsal.

Don't f*** it up the day before

If you're doing a big race, you're going to be met with samples of this and trial packs of that the day (and morning) before your race and we can't advise enough against sampling them there and then. There's only a very slim outside chance that you're going to pick something up that's going to make any difference to your race, other than making a huge mess of it. Treat race nutrition the same way you treat trainers (hopefully) by never ever getting new ones the day before a race. Eating something you've never had before is probably going to give you something much worse than a blister.

The dreaded runs...

Being a runner is actually an effective way of promoting and maintaining regular healthy bowel movements. Runners have also been shown to be at reduced risk of colon cancer. That's great news for your health. Yet there can be too much of a good thing! What about that relentless, tortuous, unwanted bowel urgency that can sometimes come about during running? You know the moment. We've all been there to varying degrees. Getting caught short, desperate for the toilet (and we're talking 'number twos' here) can be a real issue for some runners. Unwanted pit stops and increased bowel urgency during a run or race is a very common, often inconvenient, and sometimes highly embarrassing occurrence.

GI disruption

The jury's still out on this one and there's no definitive answer. Things affect people differently and why one person suffers might be different to another. There are a number of very plausible causes, ranging from lactose intolerance or reactions to other food sources, hydration status and irritable bowel syndrome. Perhaps the most common explanation is gastrointestinal (GI) disruption. More specifically, the GI tract requires a relatively still body and good blood supply to function properly. When you run, your body diverts blood flow away from the stomach and intestines and towards the heart and working muscles. Add to this jiggling, juggling and jostling of the contents of your stomach, high levels of physical exertion, nerves, anxiety and stress and you're creating a potential for diarrhoea disaster!

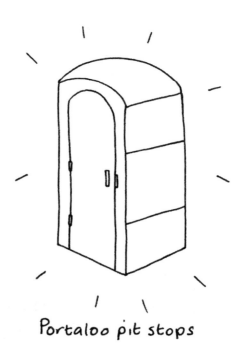

Portaloo pit stops

Don't let it put you off

Everyone is different and you'll need to experiment and find out what works best for you. Trial and correction is often the best way forwards. You might find one, a combination, or none of the suggestions below work. If you experience consistent bowel 'issues' don't be put off running altogether. Consult your GP for some specialist guidance.

The great news is that we've all been there. We are a community of oversharers and we've all got a story to tell. Master what works for you and do your best to avoid any disasters.

Tips for taming your bowels

1. Go before you go! It's the morning of the race and you're up early. Try to get used to the timings of your bowel movements so you can be prepared.

2. Establish a pre-run routine that works and helps get you 'going' before you go running.

3. Timing, type and size of pre-exercise meals. Try only eating light, low-fibre foods two to three hours before you run. Stick to simple, not rich or heavy, foods the night before your run/event.

4. Keep a food diary. Are you intolerant to some foods? Experiment with removing particular foods (dairy, wheat) from your diet and monitor what happens to your toilet habits. Find foods that work for you, especially on race day, and stick to them. Avoid trying new things or stuffing yourself at the breakfast buffet just because it's there! Avoid foods that you know give you flatulence or loose stools (dried fruit, figs, prunes, high-fibre foods).

5. Be optimally hydrated. Drink fluids but allow sufficient time for excess to pass through your system.

6. Stress, nerves and anxiety can escalate the need to evacuate! Practise keeping calm on race morning and learn some stress-busting relaxation techniques. Focus solely on your run and the things you can control.

7. Know the location of public toilets on your run routes. Sometimes friendly pub landlords, cafe owners or even shops might let you use their facilities.

8. Be environmentally sensitive if you 'go organic' in the wild. Take your paper home or bin it.

9. Try strengthening your pelvic floor muscles – these are an essential part of bowel control and help prevent leaking urine and solids.

WHY THE WALL ISN'T INEVITABLE AND BONKING ISN'T FUN

If you're training for a marathon or longer for the first time, you might have heard of something called The Wall. This mythical structure is often talked about, feared, expected. But, like all barriers, it's something you can move and have control over if you get it right. Hitting the wall or 'bonking' (more on this below) isn't inevitable, and we are going to help you avoid both.

What is the wall?

Contrary to what some believe, hitting the wall isn't something reserved for marathon runners, nor is it something you are definitely going to experience in your running. Hitting the wall, a metaphorical barrier in your race that stops you in your tracks, is usually experienced if you've got something wrong in your pre-event training, your on-the-day pacing strategy, if your nutrition isn't right or, most likely, a combination of these. The wall looks different to anyone who hits it, yet is characterised by a significant reduction in energy levels, muscular pain, a definitive drop in your ability to hold pace and potentially form, and ultimately a potential for suffering, crashing and burning! It shouldn't be something you fear or expect in your race. It can definitely be prevented with good, well-planned and well-executed pre-race training, an effective race plan, and great prior and on-the-day nutrition. If you plan to succeed, you can expect to succeed, too.

You're going to increase your chances of hitting the wall if you go out too hard or mess up your race nutrition (on the day and during the race), especially if you're also running harder than your body can tolerate or is used to.

Bonking

Bonking is the physical manifestation of hitting the wall and it really isn't pretty. It presents itself in the form of completely running out of energy, coming to a standstill or drastically reducing pace. It can bring with it jelly legs, nausea, throwing up and a serious battle with your bowels. Like the wall, bonking can happen occasionally for no reason or as an effect of running in hot weather, but it's much more likely to occur if you deplete your energy stores to such an extent that you're running on empty. Bonking doesn't always spell the end of the race, though; runners in longer distances will find themselves being able to recover and come back once toilets have been visited, fuel has been taken on and after they've had time for a good bit of positive self-talk. It's just likely that if you end up bonking in a half marathon or shorter, you're going to miss out on a positive race experience. Like the wall, bonking is entirely avoidable and in your control if you have good planning and well-practised nutrition.

It can happen to the best of us. Martin just about remembers wobbling, swaying from side to side, having goosebumps, not sweating in 35°C (95°F) heat, hallucinating, vomiting and urinating at the same time (yeah, sorry!) along the Queen K Highway in the final stages of the marathon during the World Ironman Championships in Hawaii. So we can tell you from experience: not getting it right really isn't much fun.

POST-RACE NUTRITION

Recovery fuel is something you also need to look at, not just to get through the days following your hard workouts or races more comfortably, but also to get the most from your training. You should aim to eat within 20 minutes of finishing your run, taking in something nutritious rather than a quick and sugar-heavy treat, which might be what you're secretly craving. Getting fuel on board in this window is super important in recovery, as Anji has found following a few marathons where she felt the effects of bonking hours after she'd crossed the finish line. On more than one occasion, Anji suffered a spell of post-race nausea and found eating difficult, and therefore decided to skip it completely until much later in the evening. This had a less-than-desired effect, leaving her rolled up in a ball on the bathroom floor with horrible stomach cramps, sickness and dizziness. Not the way to celebrate the end of a marathon journey! You don't need to overcomplicate this part of your routine with something expensive that promises you the world, just look to everyday options such as milkshakes, malt loaf and cereals often mentioned by runners at the top of their game.

As we've stressed throughout, nutrition is a huge foundation of you, and you as a runner. You can nourish your achievements in running by learning about fuelling and unlocking a potential secret to success. There are so many parts of nutrition that you have to personalise, and this chapter has probably given you a lot to think about. We really want you to see how important great fuelling is to your performance – cultivating your progress – as well as to your health and, above all of that, your happiness. You need to play around, experiment, practise and personalise much of what you need to race and get the most out of your training. It's a vital part of the process, and definitely one in which you can find a lot of joy.

SIX

RACE DAY

PUTTING IT ALL INTO PRACTICE

It's race day. Race day is what you've been waiting for. The time has come for you to measure your progress against yourself, your friends, your nemeses and the clock. It's time to see if you're closer to whatever goal you set yourself; even if it is just an arbitrary second, minute or hour, we know it's more than that. We know race days matter. Race day is the glorious day when you're going to see your hard work and dedication deliver. Racing makes us feel part of something much bigger, it puts us right in the heart of our community. It's the time to put into practice everything you've been learning, building, strengthening and developing. It's the time to walk the talk, to silently get the job done, to concentrate, to suffer, to succeed, to fall short, it's the time to talk to running race friends you've just met, to help them along where they need it, and to shed a few tears if it all comes together. Race day is a celebration. It's exhilarating, emotional and is always worth it (well, almost).

We are going to show you how to really engage in the process of race day to seek the outcomes that define the success you're after. You might be a serial racer with heaps of experience, but nevertheless the reminders about your head space, why you're doing it and even how to get your act together when you think you've got it nailed but still leave gaps, will prove invaluable. On the flip side, you might be a first-time racer looking for reassurances and race day tips. We've got your back.

Even with the best preparation and planning, race days can still be incredibly confusing affairs. In this chapter, we will take you through getting your head together, getting your practical things together, committing to a bit of race day suffering, enjoyment and passion, plus learning the best ways to reflect on the amazing and challenging experiences that await.

Racing is something that really allows you to engage in process and reflection. Process is what you have been through long before race day. It's the conversations with your coach and the people you run with, the training sessions that went well and the training you didn't enjoy quite as much, the rehab exercises you did for a little while and probably didn't keep up, and every single parkrun you smashed having started off thinking you were going to take it easy. We know it's good to have targets. It's good to have an end point, a goal. It's quite nice to have a medal and your name in a list of results, too. We put a lot of work into achieving targets. There are times when blood, sweat and tears go into our races, and that's how we know it really matters.

So, why are you doing this?

Chances are, you are going to ask yourself that question a lot, especially if your race is a biggie for you. Whys get defined early on, before hows and whens. Whys can change too. Is your key objective to complete, or to compete? Ask yourself this question more than once. Complete or compete? Delving deep into your why helps you turn up the heat when you need to, appreciate your race aspirations and understand how to develop your race strategy.

Beginner's whys can be far in the past by the time we have reached the midpack. While we might want to get fitter or faster over a distance or an event, we are not just getting started from scratch so fitness may not be your key why. You could be racing to raise money for a charity that's close to your heart, for a goal time you never thought was possible when you started, to do something to make your children proud, to beat your mates, to celebrate togetherness, to run in an event you've always dreamed of doing.

You're a runner, so you already know race day is amazing. It's a thing on your calendar, and you usually know the date without checking.

It's often the first thing you mention when someone asks you how you're doing. 'I'm OK, tired, training for X'. Midpack racing is the rare opportunity to share the line with champions. Now, a champion could be those speedy types at the front, but it's also every runner around us whom we celebrate with on race day. The inspiring, digging-in, working-hard, giving-it-all midpackers. You can't have a five-a-side football match with your friends on the same pitch as Manchester United while they play at the same time, but you can line up a little way behind a world record holder and run the same streets at the same time at your own pace. Whether or not you're a real athletics fan who knows and cares who those people are, that's pretty cool.

Race day is something of a carnival when you do a Big One. People are out in the streets willing you on, calling your name and giving you their complete admiration. Race day is awesome because at the same time as you're busting a gut, watching your splits, saying your mantras and counting down your distance markers, you're sometimes running on streets that are usually reserved for traffic or simply somewhere you'd never usually be at 9 a.m. on a Sunday. Racing gives you a passport to new places and with new people.

Race day is uncertain, unexpected and exciting. Despite our most amazing planning and preparation, it can throw up wonderful surprises. It's thrilling. We love race day because you never really know what's going to happen. Race day can chew you up, spit you out or give you the greatest experience of your life. Often, it's somewhere in between. You keep going back because most of the time you don't know which you'll get. It's the day when you're really going to see if it's all been worth it. You can't stop the clock on race day, you can't chuck it in and go back later and finish it off if it isn't going to plan. It strips you back, lays you bare and gives you glory or takes your heart out.

Yet, at the same time, race day almost always gives you something to celebrate. Even if you don't achieve a great result, you have a reason to celebrate the effort that went in and the resilience it took to finish. There is also a slight outside possibility that something is going to happen that means you won't finish. You can never and should never plan for this to happen, but even if you end up with the unwanted 'Did Not Finish' (DNF) by your name in the results, you're still going to know that you gave something of yourself to race day in the process of trying. You are given a free pass to tell stories, proudly wear your new race T-shirt and enjoy those weird glimmers of memories that come back to you in the following days. For those who aren't great fans of socialising, races give you ready-made excuses to leave parties early, go to bed early and take moments to be utterly selfish because you're training for the big day. You know now that training and racing at the very least gives you clarity of focus and purposeful, intentional, laser-sharp direction on a goal to be proud of.

There's so much going on in the midpack race. Not just your aspirations with regard to racing, but in the type of racing you're doing, too. We don't have the time or space in this book to break down every event from 800m on the track all the way to a multi-day, multi-stage ultra. We recognise that preparing for a trail 10k is going to look very different to preparing for your first ever attempt at 5km (3.1 miles) on the track. You know there are differences in how you feel coming to an A race that you've worked up to for three months compared to a B race you turn out for a little less prepared, and a C you go along to jog with a friend because you quite like the pie at the end. What we are going to do now is show you some of the elements of racing that are the same for you in the midpack, whatever you're working towards.

There is a lot of commonality in racing, regardless of distance, type or your aspirations. Perhaps the most fundamental is start time. The gun goes whether you are there or not. Every race will have a defined start time and if you miss that, you're screwed. There's always an element of timing or position, fellow competitors, someone faster than you, slower than you, a finish line and there's always a next time. It follows, then, that some racing strategy and planning should look the same, too, whether that's your mental preparation beforehand, how you train, pacing your race or how you reflect on it all afterwards before you go for it again.

REACHING RACE DAY

The good news about race day is that 99 per cent of the graft and hard work is behind you. Most of the mountain has been climbed. It's just the peak left to summit. Instead of having that blank training diary or empty bank of stats in your hand, you have all the training in your legs. You are no longer looking ahead to those early starts, hundreds of loads of washing, painful blisters, whatever new niggle today will bring ... you've just got today to get through. One final push. One final surge. One big celebration.

It's something of a cliché but it's true that race day is the glory lap of everything that's come before. Now is the time to truly engage with what you have done and trust the process. It's absolutely vital to trust the training you've banked. To relax in the miles you've run. To be cool with where you're at and to be up for giving it a go. Sometimes, this can be a challenge when you're surrounded by uncertainty, doubtful you've done enough, missed some miles or had a few bumps and bruises en route. Dealing with this, pressing into your learned, trialled, tested and refined psychological strategies will help you move through the midpack. Trusting your training as race day draws closer means allowing yourself the space to be where you're at. You simply cannot do any more. It is done. Now it's time to execute. Reflect on the work you put in and gain some confidence from it. There is zero adaptation to come from race day.

The type of race you are participating in will have (or certainly should have) shaped, influenced and guided your training and preparation for it, and it also helps to define your approach to race day itself.

Training for, and racing in, different kinds of running events (track racing, road racing, 5k, 10k, half marathons, ultra distance events, multi-day events, cross country, trail and mountain) varies tremendously. Preparation requires specificity (*see* Chapter 4) and racing also requires specifics, context and strategy. Our focus here sits with helping you move through the midpack in 10k to marathon participation events.

Whatever your choice of event type, personal motivations and aspirations, if you want to move through the midpack and have a great race then there are some common ground fundamentals to get right.

Reaching your best when it matters most – the taper

You're going to need to taper. Tapering is the reduction in training that comes before race day that – depending on your personality type, and how training generally went – you're going to be really excited about, or you're going to dread.

What works in the taper is different for different people and different events. There isn't a single golden tapering rule but there are some fundamental tapering basics. Essentially, a taper should see you arrive at race day fresh, energised, vibrant, motivated, focused, feeling strong, confident, competent, relaxed and ready to produce what is required for your race to turn out just as you'd hoped it would. Remember the importance of process here, though. It's no good spending months focused on the process and then throwing the baby out with the race bathwater and forgetting everything you've devoted to learning and living when race day arrives.

Tapering means running less to achieve more when it matters. This doesn't mean do nothing. It means maintaining the frequency of your running routine but dropping the volume. Include some shorter, higher-intensity workouts and some paced efforts, depending on what you're aiming for in your race. Make sure as the race draws closer you feel fresh and recovered and not tired. The very best you can do for yourself and for race day is to tick over

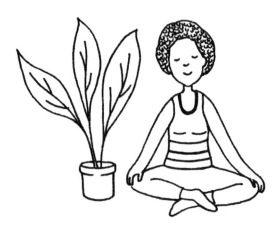

Tapering ; relaxed readiness to perform.

and become a coiled spring that's ready to pop when the time is right. The worst thing you can do is keep going as you were, feel knackered and arrive at your start line with an injury.

If you normally run three or four times a week then keep that regular routine going right up until race week but run for a shorter duration and cut the volume of both your individual workouts and your weekly total. Running volume, and again that's both person and event specific, or running super hard, or doing tons of high-intensity training the week before the race will only serve to tire you out before you've even started your race. Typically, think about it in terms of reducing your volume by 30 per cent of your weekly total running three weeks out, 60 per cent two weeks out and 90 per cent with one week to go.

Having a great taper is important to having a great race because tapering/reducing your training allows your body to get to a state of feeling fresher and your mind to a point of focus. It's all about readiness to perform at your best. Midpack runners have lives, and jobs and responsibilities so it's quite easy to just stick to routine and carry on regardless. 'It's Tuesday! I do track on Tuesday!' Routine is great, but it's important to get the balance right. Spending 10 days doing absolutely nothing before your race isn't going to come easy to a midpack runner who's dedicated X amount of weeks to achieving X goal, but like many things in running, tapering is quite a personal thing, too. Great tapering is also learned, event specific, situational, related to experience and individual. What works for one runner in a taper may well not work for another. For example, some runners prefer a 'shallow' gradual taper, started from weeks out with a steady reduction in volume, while others prefer a steep or sharp taper leaving a more significant drop until the final few days. Trialling and testing in cardboard box races is how you'll learn what works for you so you can execute your best personal strategy for your Big One.

Tapering is done best when it involves an element of self-preservation, but without you becoming an anxious hermit for three weeks before your big day. You don't need to hide away and bubble wrap your body but you do need to be aware of looking after yourself. Don't fall into the trap of filling the time you'd usually be out running longer on a Sunday with a high-risk DIY activity you've been putting off for ages. Similarly, new adventurous hobbies can wait. Rock climbing, BMX stunt practice and even the wholesome-looking online squat challenge you've been tagged in should wait until race day is over. Spend the time instead working out where you're going to park or what the nearest pub is likely to have on the menu when you get there at the end.

Tapering is the time for you to trust the training you've done and let your body adapt to the miles you've covered. You won't lose any of the fitness you have gained over the past few months by being sensible and doing less as the race draws closer. Fitness adaptations take time. The benefits of regular, appropriate and progressive training are realised in fitness and form weeks and months after the actual training has been completed. Although fitness takes a while to build up it also takes a while to lose (although not as long). By staying active during your taper, including the same frequency of runs, including a little intensity but dropping the duration, you maintain your fitness and stamina while also ensuring that you're fully refreshed and recovered to hit race day.

Golden rules for a cracking taper

1. Back off and do less. Resist the temptation to run more miles. Run smart. Don't look at what anyone else is doing. This is all about you.

2. Eat a healthy, well-balanced and nutrient-dense diet. That doesn't mean you need to stuff your face at the pre-race pasta party. A reduction in training volume coupled with an adequate fuel intake should optimise your energy stores. Don't try anything new.

3. Even though you might have a little more time, don't fill your taper period with extra jobs or overcommit socially or to work. Leave the DIY until after the race! Reduce work stress if you can, too; now is not the time to work towards the deadlines you've been repeatedly putting off.

4. Remind yourself of all the good things you've achieved in your training over the past few months and see yourself running a strong race.

5. Get an extra hour's sleep each night in the week leading up to the race.

COUNTDOWN TO RACE DAY

21 days to go
- Sharp running that is at target pace. Know what this is. Master it.
- Last longer run (for marathon distance and over). Start to ease it back.
- Mental prep started or in flow (remember, you should have been putting this is place throughout your training build-up and not have left trying it out until the taper).

14 days to go
- Last longer run (for races shorter than marathon).
- Mental prep in full flow. Know it. Practise it.
- Logistical planning started.

7 days to go
- Enter taper mode! Reduced volume, reduced intensity.
- Comfortable, easy running most of the time.
- Dress rehearsal covered in the mind – walk through what you are wearing, where you will start, what time you need to leave etc.
- Race plan created, including key splits and plans for tough moments.

5 days to go
- Last faster workout completed.
- Full lead-in kit check completed, including any fuel needed for race day (nothing new!).
- Mental check-in. Revise the race plan and test yourself on elements of it.

3 days to go
- Check your race information again. Know your start times, start zone, where the nearest toilets are.
- Check in with anyone you are relying on for race day.

- Using your kit inventory from earlier in the week, pack all your kit. Lay it out and double-check everything. If you're not sure whether or not to take something then take it – it's better to have it and not want it.
- Do a short easy run. Just run, don't think, don't stress.

2 days to go
- This might be your last chance for normal sleep, so get an extra hour today if you can.
- Reflect again on your race plan.
- Eat well – be fuelled and hydrated. No need to overeat.
- Rest or go for a very short, very easy run.

1 day to go
- It's almost here! Don't eat anything new, different or 'special spicy'!
- Do a flat lay. Lay out all of your kit for tomorrow right down to socks and trainers. Pin your race number on now so you're not rushing around looking for pins in the morning.
- Do a breakfast flat lay. Before you go to bed, make sure you have everything laid out ready for breakfast.
- Get your self-talk together. Talk kindly to yourself. Reframe any thoughts you're having about tomorrow positively. Build an 'I can do this' mindset.
- Relax and be kind to yourself. Go for a short walk, listen to music, read a book, take a bath. Do any of the things that make you feel good.
- Remember...
  1. Stick to what you know. Nothing new, ever.
  2. Be organised and prepped. Know your route, timings, travel.
  3. Chill, rest, reflect and stay calm.
  4. Enjoy. Enjoy escaping routine – find a new normal.

RACE DAY PSYCHOLOGY – 'HOW'S YOUR TRAINING GONE?'

You're on the start line, you turn and your fellow racer blurts out: 'How's training gone, what's your plan today'? Gulp. You turn away, pausing as you search for the right/best/only answer. Many runners might be tempted at this point to fire back with a wishy-washy excuse as to why they have reached race day not as fit as they'd like because of that injury, that bug, that busy job, that broken toe, those missed miles or that dog that ate their trainers. Whatever.

Lie. You're there now. It's not changing. Be ready.

Most midpack runners have had that 'why do I do this to myself?' feeling on race day. Racing isn't all punching the air and floating over finish lines feeling equally triumphant and spent. Sometimes racing is nerve-wracking. Racing makes us nervous because, ultimately, this is a very public test with a very wide audience. If you're someone who allows nerves to sabotage your races, you will know how destructive (and self-fulfilling) they can be. But we think that nerves are important and positive as they get us jumping up and down at start lines exploding with energy minutes before we cross the timing mats. Nerves remind us that racing is important to us. It's what we came for.

Reasons for racing will widely vary from person to person in the midpack. We want to get fitter, we want to run faster, we want to go further. We want our running to take us to new places emotionally, geographically, physically, even for some spiritually, too. Racing is to some extent expected of us. 'You training for anything then?' carries with it something of a loaded question – they're probably also wondering how fast you're going to run it, too.

We already know racing gives us focus, especially when it follows a hefty dose of focused training. Race day is there for us to come together with everyone like us in a beautiful, exhausting display of the thing we love to do. Race day is for our stories, for our 'why', it's our big display of effort, the time to show off our best gear, our fancy dress and our personal challenges.

Nail it! Reach race day remembering to:

1. Draw on your nerves. Understand them. See them as energy to fuel your race.
2. Know your why. Remind yourself about your purpose, passion and vision for your race. It's now that it matters the most.
3. Get ready to focus. Understand what this truly means, how you can activate your focus, how you can switch it on and off, turn it up and down. It's time to put in place all that you practised in your training build-up. Know what focus tools you can bring out from your armoury, and when and how to apply them before and during your race.

Race day is the time to concentrate

Concentration means locking into your race day task. When you concentrate, your mind stays focused, you can apply yourself with purpose, clarity and focus. Without distraction, in the right ways at the right times. Concentration needs to happen before race day, on race morning and during the race. At the same time, you don't need to be super intense with your concentration strategy. It's really hard to concentrate with true intention and deep capacity for prolonged periods of time. If your race is of a longer duration, understanding how to dial your concentration up and down, to level it up or to relax it, is a vital part of the race execution process. Intense concentration at the wrong time can lead to unwanted anxiety and badly timed pressure points. This can jeopardise race day and risk you concentrating on the wrong things (such as how 'bad'/slow/out of shape/off pace you feel) at the wrong time and inevitably risk race day collapse. The trick is to understand what works for you and when and how to use it.

You might be someone who never listens to music when they race, but will always take music and audiobooks on training runs. Some feel that listening to music, especially when racing, cheats them out of the experience of hearing hundreds of pairs of feet hit the road around them, or a voice in the crowd cheering them on. Some are helped along by cheering and encouragement from spectators. Others, though, may need to get in the zone with their own soundtracks to drown anything else out. You will know which camp you fall into. Paul Tonkinson sums this up in his book *26.2 Miles to Happiness*, writing: 'Not to be too crude, though it fits the mood, the crowd were getting on my tits. Their cries of encouragement fell hollow in my ears,' as he struggled his way through a bad patch during the London Marathon.

Concentrating in a race is really important even if you're not going for a specific time. Race day gives you a list of new variables that you've rarely had to deal with in training. Bigger races may have curve balls in the shape of discarded potential ankle-breakers such as bottles, lids and gel packets, people pulling up and stopping ahead of you, and a racing line you can't really see. There are a lot of us in the midpack and it isn't always easy to tell if we are following the most direct path to the finish.

Concentrating is also vital if you want to get your pacing right. 'Right' doesn't always mean achieving a specific time. It can mean just not going off so hard that you blow to pieces and crawl home miserably. Real concentration when it comes to pacing shouldn't always include a heavy reliance on GPS – in fact, in big-city racing this is a really bad idea. Huge groups of people in one place with tall buildings, tunnels and bridge crossings will mean your GPS is at some stage likely to go wrong. Reliance on GPS means you will very probably end up flapping every time you reach a physical distance marker because the chances are your watch lied to you and told you you'd reached it a few minutes ago. We don't suggest going naked without a watch, just prepare to concentrate later in your race when you might need some PB maths to work out your splits using time elapsed and distance markers.

It's also good to focus on you as much as you can. This is *your* moment. Losing concentration can lead to falling into someone else's pace. It's a bad thing if they're too fast for you because you're going to blow up and regret it, and it's also a bad thing if they're too slow for you because you're going to fall short and regret it. Locking in with someone running the exact same pace is rare and wonderful when it happens and it's the stuff lifelong friendships are made of, so make sure you take note of their race number at the finish…

Concentrate and nail it!

1. Know when to switch on and off your concentration.
2. Keep your high-intensity concentration limited to focused periods.
3. Concentrate on different things at different times.
4. Relax into concentration. Settle your emotions.

LOGISTICS AND ORGANISATION – 'IT'S TIME TO GET YOUR SHIT TOGETHER'

Be organised before race day hits. Without wishing to sound like a nagging parent, if you haven't grasped the basics of your personal admin and organisation then race day will break you (if you make it at all!).

Your physical training and mental prep mean nothing without effective logistical planning. This is true of any race you ever do. It's time to get your shit together. If you're always late, now is the time to buck the trend. Don't be someone chasing after the baggage truck or pinning your race number on as you cross the start mat. Trust us, that just causes unwanted stress and anxiety.

Successful race logistics are just as important as training in reducing the stress you can't avoid on race day. Don't get complacent just because you've done this so many times before. We have heard of people training diligently for months for races that they then go on to miss completely because they misread the start time. So be just as diligent in checking your race information, your kit and the tried-and-tested positive elements of your training routine. The last few days should signal a reduction in training, giving you the time to get this stuff right.

The final few hours before the race are just as important. You need to do everything you can to minimise stress and that includes allocating time to do things that need a bigger time budget than you're used to. Yes, we mean toilet queues. This is the time when your race logistics really matter and that includes getting warmed up and ready to go. You will either be a talker or someone who needs to avoid contact with everyone. Get your last bits of nutrition right, and that's especially important if you're running a longer distance. We know now your race nutrition should be nailed and effective, so don't muff it up by being tempted by a sample of whatever is on offer in the car park from the race sponsor (shove it in your bag to try out at another time, if you like). You need to minimise the risk of seeing anything again a few miles down the road.

It's really important to have your post-race shit together too. At bigger races, there may be a wait for your bag, then a wait for your friends, then another wait for transport. Think through the possibilities and make sure you take what you need. Don't get caught out on something that will impact your recovery in the first few hours after finishing – you're going to have enough to think about!

Getting it nailed:

1. Be on time (or early) for everything.
2. Nothing new ever. Again.
3. Have the right stuff waiting in your bag for you at the end.

How to plan a race strategy

Here are five really important questions to ask yourself before race day:

1. What does this race mean to you?
2. What would you like to achieve in this race?
3. What are you confident you could do to execute this race well?
4. Define your race process. What are you going to do, when? How are you going to approach this race?
5. What mental strategies do you know work for you and when are you going to deploy them for optimal effect in this race? (What will you do when it's going right, and wrong?)

RACE CRAFT AND RACE PLANS

You learn to race. It's called developing your race craft. It only comes with practice. Inherent in this practice is getting it wrong. A lot. A part of improving your midpack performance is to unpack your race craft, your learned race skills, and rearrange them in such a way that they work for you. With more experience, more mistakes, more learning, you'll build a race day formula that sees your training, tapering and race craft be realised in the execution of the 'perfect race'. These will be the races that you remember most (alongside the total shockers!). They'll be the priceless finish lines where you've gutted yourself, rinsed yourself, turned yourself inside out to break that stubborn PB that's been evading you for years. When your desire to run well, to break barriers, to achieve more than you ever thought you could has long left you and you're recounting your running highlights, your show reel, your lifetime, standout races that made you, a small but not insignificant number of personal performances will strike at the forefront of your memory with power and clarity. Cherish these memories. The days when the sun shone, when you got it all right, it all went to plan and you bathed in the warm glory of success and the cold metal of the finishers' medal swung around your neck for a week! Great races that are etched on your memory won't always be the ones that go well. Some of our 'best' races are complete horror stories. However, your chances of having a race to remember are greatly increased by learning your race day trade and practising your race craft. Learning to race, planning to race, executing that final push is what makes your races matter. Planning to get race day right helps you to realise the outcomes you're after.

Race plans and how to get one

Having a race plan simply means not pitching up without a clue what you're doing. Seriously, take it from us, you'll be gutted if you prepare super diligently for the 'race of your life' and then bowl up having not planned your approach to the race. When you've thought it through, you're more able to stay calm, to focus your attention, to give your energy to running well, to execute it with a intentionality, to flex and give when it doesn't go to plan, to work with wobbles (because you've thought them through, and the last time you cocked it up you paid the price big time!), to survive when you need to and attack when you can.

Despite having the best-laid race plans, they can, do and will go wrong. When that happens, don't completely throw in the towel. Having quality race craft is about expecting the unexpected, being comfortable with discomfort and being certain in times of uncertainty. It's just a fact that races can throw things at you when you're not expecting them – a delayed start, torrential rain, the biggest headwind in the history of headwinds, a fall, a trip, a diversion, pain, suffering, anger and frustration. You can choose to respond brilliantly, work through tough times, apply practised strategies, respond, adapt, be agile, commit and press on and be rewarded with a magical race day memory. At other times, it all just goes wrong, you have no idea why, but you scrape yourself up and live to fight and run another day.

Race plans can be developed as race day draws closer. Sometimes you won't know the specifics of your approach until race week. Form can change, illness can occur, injuries can creep up on you, you can feel fitter and be faster than you thought. Developing your race strategy is a personal thing that takes trial and error.

SUCCESSFUL RACE PLANNING: WHAT DO YOU WANT TO ACHIEVE AND HOW WILL YOU DO IT?

- Plan your race pace strategy – even splits, royal flush (each section faster), negative split (second half faster), taking into account the course profile. Seriously, mess this up in the first miles and you've blown it. Prepare yourself for a suffer-fest. Control yourself! This is really simple: don't go off like a rocket at the start.
- Learn your nutrition strategy – what you need to eat before, during and immediately after the race. If you are eating during the race, know at which distance or time you need each 'feed' and be clear on them, they can be easy to forget in later stages when they are actually most important.
- Nail your hydration strategy – when you are planning to drink, with good knowledge of where drinks stations are and what they offer (check if they use bottles, cups or pouches, too).
- Plan for possible issues and scenarios encountered and how to deal with them. The main thing to remember is that you are in control of how you react to whatever the race throws at you. It is very rare for a race to go completely to plan.

You might run a long course, you could hit an unexpected headwind or get a stitch, or you might miss a water station. Unless you end up injured or ill, you are still going to finish, but you have to remain in control to deal with those moments in between. Your calm reactions to them really matter. You can't change what happens, you can only change your reactions.

- Know your start spot and choose where you go from. This is easier in smaller races but work out where you are going to feel best – even if that's within a corral. This doesn't mean you need to elbow your way to the front, but it also may not mean standing right at the back and being faced with a wall of runners from the off. Find runners who are aiming to finish in a similar time to your goal and run at your pace and stick with them.

- Know the route. Course maps will be available online for weeks if not months ahead of the race. Get advice from people who have run it before on where are the best places to kick, where you might need to back off, and things such as bottlenecks and hills that might come as a surprise otherwise. Understand sections where you need to concentrate, work hard and be strong, and sections where you can relax and stride out.

- Run evenly. Depending on the length of your race, chunks of distance should be easy for you to work towards. Whether you run them in 1 mile (1.6km) chunks, 5km (3.1-mile) chunks or you're expecting to run for days, work out a plan using what you know about the course to inform what pace you plan to run each chunk at, and make them as even as possible.

- The last chunk is supposed to hurt! Plan for this discomfort and how you are going to deal with it. If you've got your pacing right and are in with a shout of your PB within the final chunk, then remember that slowing down at this point isn't an option! The final section can make all the difference so finish strong and smiling.

Control the controllables

You have to start by trying to put aside all the things you can't control. Everyone is guilty to an extent – even if you're just frantically weather checking, you're trying to change or control something that is none of your business. It's time for you to focus on what you can control, and that includes the preparation that happens in the last few days before the race. To an extent, you can control what you eat, your sleep routine, how much time you spend on your feet. It's totally OK if there are interruptions to these if you're going to race further away from home, but again just control what you can. Getting your practical stuff together is part of this.

That start line feeling is pretty amazing. We are lucky in the midpack because we sometimes get a precious few extra minutes – especially at big races – to cross the start line. It's where you can take a few seconds to wish a fellow midpacker luck, wish yourself luck, take a deep breath, take it all in. The moment you're been counting down to is actually here. The only thing you have to remind yourself is to keep control of that opening part of the race ahead, those early miles; letting go of all that built-up excitement and nervous energy is important to the rest of your race.

Racing 'well' – whatever that looks like to you – begins with having a strategy. It really depends on the type of race you're doing and knowing what you want to get out of it. People often struggle in races when the plan for the race itself isn't clear, or you haven't been sure where to start in building one. If you're not clear on how to execute your race, your confidence is going to wobble, and every race will, in some way, have a different strategy, whether that's because you have to survive over long, multiple days in an ultra or you've got to cope with the uncomfortable eyeballs-out feeling of running something short and hard on a track.

MASTER YOUR MINDSET

Race day is all about facing fears, controlling the things that are in your control, harnessing nerves and anxiety positively, overcoming adversity, developing empowering self-belief. Most of all, it's about staying in control so you don't mess up when it really comes down to it.

You know what you've spent the last few months working on and what you want to achieve. You don't need to prepare a poem to recite to yourself in the mirror – those tiny mirrors in race day toilets are much too small for that. But it might help you to have something of a mantra. Try to go with something sharp that reminds you why you're doing this, that you can do it, you are ready. Some people in the midpack take confidence from reminding themselves of all the training that went to plan and everything they ticked off on the way. Others do the opposite, preferring to draw on the runs and workouts that they found particularly hard. It can be reassuring to think back to a particularly demanding session that you never thought you'd get through, and did. Your mental preparation should include a pep talk that features whatever it takes to put you in a positive and attacking frame of mind.

Whether you think you can, or you think you can't, you're right. Apply this to your racing head. If you spend the days and weeks leading up to your big day imagining your success or seeing the time you want on the clock, it's more likely to happen and give you a positive mindset for racing. It follows, then, that thinking negative thoughts and imagining scenarios in which things go wrong means that they are more likely to happen, too. It's really important that you don't leave this stuff too late, either. It's just as important as ticking off your hard workouts and training sessions that you take some time to practise getting your head right. Ask yourself, what do you want from your race day? You know the why and through your training you should also know the how. Look back at all of the tips we gave you in Chapter 2. It's too late to start thinking about those tricks and tips for a good running mindset the night before the race when you have too many other logistical bits to consider. These should have been the backbone of your psychological pre-race preparation. By the time race day hits, you should know these inside out. You will know how twitchy racing makes you and you're likely to know by now how that will manifest itself. If you're someone who can harness nerves into excitement, this is a great positive exercise to try to bring to your training and plough into some really fantastic workouts. Reflecting on how you feel when things go well is really powerful, too.

Try adding workouts and scenarios into your training that bring about a little controlled but manageable twitchiness in your build-up, whether that's something that will make you uncomfortable (running a very short, easy run on a day you'd expect something long and fast) or something that will test your resilience (running a loop that goes right past your front door several times without stopping over a long distance, for example). Pitch you against you, wrestle the tension and develop your controlled response. If you're smart about this, you know what makes you twitchy and with planning and training you can add these elements to your build-up in the same way you do with your workouts. It's about getting your head together when things feel uncomfortable and putting yourself in that scenario through the process of your training as many times as you can so that race day feels a little less daunting. Fail to prepare your head in the same way you prepare your body, though, and you're probably going to muff it up. It's a key part of learning race craft and mastering a really great race.

THIS IS GOING TO HURT

If you want to hit your race right out of the park you are going to have to get out of your comfort zone to achieve something amazing. If a result in your Big One is what's driving you, you won't be able to slide on your comfy shoes and glide without some time in the hurt locker. Getting something special out of race day is probably going to get uncomfortable. Be ready to bring that on, absorb it, turn it your advantage. Prepare yourself for the fact that race day is going to hurt and that you're OK with that. Being able to identify, spend time in, work through the locker without letting it get the better of you is an important element of moving through the midpack. The great news is it's also a lived experience thing that can be embraced rather that feared. The locker is an uncomfortable space you're going to climb in and out of, possibly multiple times. Maybe you're going to get into it and stay there, but you can handle it. Your physical training and mental preparation should reassure you that it's OK to hurt! You are still in control despite the breathlessness, the fatigue, the soreness, the doubt. Even if your goal really is just to 'get round' you're still likely to have moments when your brain and body go into battle, so you need to go into racing with an element of acceptance. Tell yourself, it's OK to hurt and it's going to be OK. You're in control of the discomfort. You have been here before. You can notice it hurts, but let it pass. It will pass. Patiently sit with the discomfort, embrace it and come to terms with it.

This is suffering. This is racing. This is running beyond your potential. This why you are here. This is moving through the midpack.

In longer distance or duration events, you might hit a point where you feel like you have nothing left. You might experience 'the wall' (*see* p. 156), in which case it's very likely you'll get a second wind if you manage to get some fuel on board. But you might also 'just' mentally get to the point of feeling like you have nothing left. Spoiler – yes you have. Everyone has something in them (usually at the sight of the finish line) that is there to keep them going, it's just another of the great mysteries of running. Keep reminding yourself that nothing lasts forever. In fact, one of the best things about running, especially longer distances, is that you can come back and feel better multiple times. It's unlikely a rough patch will last the whole way, and you know that from your training. Trust your training. Tough moments arrive and they will pass. Work through them. Focus on the footstep in front of you and only that. Run the mile you are in. Again, we are going to harp on about process here; trust the process of everything you put into your training to arrive at race day and give yourself the best possible chance of getting through it. So, here it is again:

1. It's going to hurt. Learn to engage, embrace and be comfortable with that.
2. Have a comeback strategy for when you feel like you're losing it.
3. Trust the process, trust the process, trust the process.
4. Wherever you think the edge is, you can learn to spend more time there than you think is possible.

All that said, of course you need to know and understand the difference between bravado, ego and just plain silliness. There are important signals your body sends your brain when it's feeling fatigued and although we can teach ourselves to gain a better understanding and awareness of these so that we can push at the right times when it matters most, we should also teach ourselves to know when today isn't our day.

There are, of course, times when we should know how and when to listen to the sensory signals our body and brain sends us. Knowing when to stop is as important as knowing when to push. It's also important to learn to understand through experience how your body feels and responds and in doing so be really in tune when something doesn't feel really right. Knowing your own personal history is very important. Using this history, your training knowledge, your form knowledge and an accurate judgement of your personal safety and health, you can learn to work with discomfort but you shouldn't push through acute, intense, sudden or surprising pain. Know when to back off. Know when slowing down and stopping is sensible, advisable and necessary.

HOW TO NAIL YOUR RACE

Not all races are created equal and gearing yourself for a race will be different depending on what you know about yourself, your preparation, your aspirations, your motivations, your ability and what you know about the race. Objectives for racing can vary considerably. How you approach one race can be very different to how you approach another one, depending on where it fits in your training and racing cycle (*see* Chapter 4), the terrain, type and distance. One thing that's pretty fixed about race types, though, is the event distance. We're going to share some pointers on how to tackle 5k, 10k, half marathon and marathon racing.

Going faster – racing 5k

A 5km (3.1-mile) run might be over pretty quickly (quickly is a relative term!) but most of you will know the glory of what it's like to get them just right. These races and parkruns are brilliant to use as a tune-up to something longer, as a hard threshold workout in place of a session or as a standalone time trial. Thanks to the global success of parkrun, we all know what our 5k bests are, and probably what we want them to be, too!

In a 5k, you have to be prepared to hit the gas as soon as the gun goes. Perhaps in 5k, more than other events, that makes it super important that you get a good warm-up in to ensure you're stoked and ready to fire. You can't expect to go from 0–5k pace without a little pre-race tune up. Make sure as you head to the start that you're in the right place in the pack so you can get straight into your personal pace and don't leave yourself too much to catch up.

You need to get psyched to run fast. A 5k race demands a mindset shift. To get a fast 5k, you've really got to get your head and heart into the hurt locker. The effort level is high and you've got to get mentally geared up for fast running and high performance. Learning to concentrate in fast, short racing like this helps you concentrate in longer running, too.

In longer-distance races you have more time to get into the run and it's more about being sensible, sometimes backing off and pacing yourself at the start. In a 5k, you've got less time to think and plan. It's much more about higher percentage effort and hanging on to a faster pace from the get-go. If you get it wrong and start too quickly, you've not got that long to hang on and you learn a great deal about your top-end threshold speed and how it feels to manage faster running. Try to run even kilometre splits for the first 3km (1.9 miles), then gradually start to chip away as you wind it up into the last 2km (1.2 miles) so you can finish strong. The best 5k times are run when it starts to feel like agony as you hang on for glory at the finish. Use others ahead of you as targets to reach and pass. Focus on your form, get it done and leave it all on the course.

Getting stronger – racing 10k

The right mindset for a 10k is a strong one. You know it's going to hurt, especially in the second half, and you need to be ready for this.

Before the race start, stay calm. Thoroughly complete a warm-up routine that works for you. It needs to physically and psychologically prepare you for what's to come. Roll over in your head your race strategy, fight any doubts away and go over your race scenarios. Keep that belief in your ability to execute your plan. You've done the training and are ready. Positively visualise your success. See yourself running strongly and achieving your goals.

It's natural to have a wobble during the race and start to doubt your ability to make the finish but at the same time you've got to commit. To run a great 10k, you can't spend the first half of the race gently getting into it. You've got to be hitting your target race pace quickly and focusing on holding it for each kilometre. Break the 10km (6.2 miles) down into 10 x 1km or 6 x 1 miles and focus only on hitting your desired time for each unit. Tick them off mentally.

Start off fast but not crazy fast and find your 10k target pace within the first mile. A great 10k requires you to settle down and get into a smooth rhythm during the first two miles, so you can continue to feel controlled and strong. Take inspiration from those around you and get into a pack if you can. Between miles 4 and 5 (6.4–8km), block out distractions. Tune into your body and how you are feeling in order to stay on pace. Concentrate really hard as it starts to really hurt. As you approach the final mile, remind yourself that you are doing what you've done in training (we know we make it sound easy when we say it like that), that you are strong, have the ability to stay bang on pace and can tolerate time in the hurt locker as you roll into the final ¼ mile (400m) to finish the race off. Racing 10k has to be relentless to be successful. You won't nail your 10k by being easy on yourself.

Going the distance – racing a half marathon

Running a fast half marathon is as much in the head and the heart as in the legs and lungs. Although your engine might be capable of running faster than you've run before, if your mind isn't ready to go the distance then you may stutter mid-race. You know now that much of your confidence to run fast in a race comes from confident training. Although negative thoughts may creep in mid-race when your legs are burning and your heart is pounding, remind yourself that you've been here many times in training and can handle the pressure and the pace right through to the finish. Having a strong mindset and a clear strategy will get you started positively. When things do start to hurt halfway through (or ideally at about mile 12/19.3km!) – and they will – remind yourself that you have what it takes to deliver your goal and that you're tough enough to hold your target pace. Break the final part of the race down into smaller sections.

During the first mile (1.6km) get quickly into your target half marathon race pace. Be patient. Be controlled. Be confident. There's still a long way to go. Through miles 2 to 5 (3.2–8km) settle into your running groove. Keep your pace on track (if anything, it's OK to be slightly up on pace here). Simmer and tick along in control. As you approach mile 6 (9.6km) and pass halfway into miles 7 and 8 (11.3–12.9km), it's really the time to focus. Have a pace check at the halfway mark. It's easy for your mind to wander here. Remind yourself that your best running will be done in the second half. Control the middle to two-thirds of the race. This will test your resolve, determination and training. Be disciplined and stay on pace track. You'll need to draw on your fitness at this stage to confidently control your race through halfway and head into the third quarter of the race.

Miles 9, 10 and 11 (14.5, 16 and 17.7km) are the most important part of your race. Dig deep and keep going. Staying on pace in these three miles can make or break your PB. Tick off each individual mile. It's during these miles that you'll most likely hit the premium fatigue. The stuff that shapes you as a runner. The choice moments to back off the pace and settle for letting it slide happen here. As you pass mile 10 (16km), remind yourself it's only a parkrun to go.

Finally, miles 12 and 13 (and a bit) (19.3–20.9km-plus) are the push into your final stretch. This is where you cash your money miles training cheques. It's where you stay on course with relentless confidence and drive towards the finish line or it's where you'll fold and flop and break your flow and fall off your pace. During the last 2 miles (3.2km) you'll need to trust the training you've done and push your physical and mental boundaries to deliver your race goal.

Going longer – racing a marathon

Whether it's your first or your 50th marathon, you are likely to feel very nervous at the start ... that's OK, it's a long way! Take a few minutes to calm yourself, stand confidently on the start line and reflect on all your positive moments in training and racing and how far you've come in your marathon journey.

In Martin's role as official coach to the London Marathon he's seen a lot of marathon runners, answered a lot of marathon questions, and been privileged to see some incredible marathon finishes, from world records to runners carrying washing machines, running against the odds, and challenging themselves to complete a lifetime goal in a way in which they never thought possible. Running a marathon is a tough gig. Running a marathon hard, to the best of your ability, is even tougher. When you've put all your eggs in your marathon basket and you pitch up ready to lay it all on the line, it's a day that really matters. Getting a marathon race right isn't easy. It's difficult to get everything right for 26.2 miles (42.2km) on the bounce and one thing is for certain: a marathon, when you're trying to run it hard, is going to test you to the core and throw things at you that challenge you physically and emotionally. But, when you nail that marathon race day, it sticks.

Racing a marathon well is about so much more than race day. To get it right you've got to arrive ready. Arrive poorly prepared, lacking in miles, missing some fundamentals and a marathon run hard will find you out. There is nowhere to hide at mile 20 (32km) when the wheels have come off, you're wrecked and you know you've got to suffer out the final 6 miles (9.7km) and it's going to push you beyond what's normal. But that's also the beauty and elegance of the marathon. It's a beast that will own you unless you control and own it.

Anji always promised herself she would do a marathon before she turned 40, and it came a few years before that at Liverpool in 2014, when she was 33. This happened a little by accident as she had spent a few months training with a friend she was coaching, and it got to a point where she felt that the training may as well be used for something. Somewhat frustratingly, that first marathon, still to this day, is Anji's best time. Running a marathon has always been an experience of high emotions. For example, she ran with Ben Smith in the 401 Challenge (Ben ran 401 marathons in 401 days for Stonewall and Kidscape charities) just a few weeks after her dad's death in 2016, and then again in a comeback from illness thanks to a heart condition, at the London Marathon in 2019. The marathon often represented what had once felt an impossible dream, and now with four marathons under her belt, it is a reality she is always keen for others to experience, too. This is in some ways what Anji feels is a superpower, that 'If I can do it, anyone can' story to tell.

We've both made mistakes in our marathon running. Without doubt, the number one marathon race balls-up is to think you're world record holder Eliud Kipchoge on the start line and go speeding through the first 6 miles (9.7km) way too fast. Pacing your race is the most important aspect of getting race day right. It's easy to get excited, forget the best-laid plans of starting slowly and go off too fast. Starting too fast makes running the second half of the race very tough indeed! You need to learn how to control your pace and run an even, well-paced marathon. Everyone should know their race day pace targets or risk blowing out in the final 6 miles (9.7km). Know your target pace by having a target finish time (e.g. 4 hours) and working this out as the 'pace per mile' you need to run to finish in this time. For example, 9 minutes and 9 seconds/mile (6 minutes and 15 seconds/km) equates to a 4-hour marathon finish, and 11 minutes and 27 seconds/mile (7 minutes/km) equates to a 5-hour marathon finish. Practise running at your target marathon pace in your training runs and learn how it feels. It should feel manageable, controllable and 'easy'. On race day, what feels easy after 5 miles (8km) will feel harder after 25 miles (40.2km)!

Depending on the number of runners taking part and your position within them, it might take a few minutes to cross the start line, which can make it a little difficult to control your pace right at the start. Stay calm, breathe, relax. You've got this. Be patient. Perhaps the most common mistake made by even the most experienced marathon runners is that they start too fast. Once the race starts, runners around you might be moving faster than you but stick to your pace plan as much as possible. In mass participation races during the first mile, you will likely be running very close to other runners and may find it hard to get into your running stride, especially if they are running slightly slower or faster than you want to go. Just relax and don't waste energy weaving through people or trying to keep up.

Allow your pace, breathing and stride pattern to settle down. Just tick the first few miles of the race off in a consistent, metronomic style. Use as little energy as you can as the race unfolds. Feel yourself get into your running. Once you've got the first few miles under your belt you'll ease into things, the nerves will pass and you'll find yourself flowing and ready to tackle the distance.

You'll have made your energy and fluids decisions and worked out your strategy before the race, including whether or not you will use what's there on the course or take your own. Either way, there's no need to stop at the first water/drinks station on course and neck everything available! If you're adequately hydrated before the race it doesn't matter if you skip the frenzy of the first station. Focus on your own strategy and drink to thirst, taking energy on board in the first half of the race to keep you strong in the second.

When you do reach an aid station you want to use, you don't need to rush for the first person who offers you a drink. Take your time and stay relaxed. In bigger races, there are many helpers passing you a drink and an aid station may stretch for 50–100m (55–110 yards). Often, the people towards the middle and back of the aid stations have more space and grabbing a drink from them is easier. Be patient once you have your drink. Carry it with you and sip it for a while.

Before race day, you should have reviewed the route and course and know how it's going to unfold. Break it up into landmarks, features on route, mile markers, points of interest, or spots where family of friends will be standing cheering. Once you go through mile 8 (12.9km) celebrate the fact that you'll have covered the first third of the race. This is a great milestone and one to be proud of. This first third of a marathon is so important. It can really set you up for the all-important middle and final thirds of the race. At this point, you should still be feeling comfortable and in control. Hit cruise control for the middle third of the race. One of your key marker points and stepping stones for your finish is the halfway point (13.1 miles/21km), so focus on that now. Your goal is to reach that point feeling as fresh as you can and ready to tackle the second half. Your marathon really begins here.

It's important to be disciplined and controlled but it doesn't always go to plan. What happens if you feel good but are minutes down on your target time at the halfway mark? Don't try to play catch up and smash out the next couple of miles to pull yourself quickly back on track. The best marathons are run with even splits and pacing throughout the entire race so take your time to claw back those valuable seconds mile by mile as the second half progress. This is also a good time to pay extra attention to relaxing as you progress from miles 13 to 16 (20.9–25.7km). Focus on you and how you're feeling. Tune into your body. Take time to relax, run smoothly and enjoy the moment and what you are achieving. Remind yourself how far you've come on your journey. Think about how you started your marathon campaign and enjoy the fact that this is it. You are doing it. Compose yourself and get yourself ready for the final third of the race – without doubt the toughest part.

Marathons are won or lost in the final miles and so you need to be physically and mentally braced for the battle with yourself that lies ahead. Although your effort level will be higher, your fatigue greater and the pain more intense, you've got to keep moving and keep striving to hold your even pace. This is the part of the marathon that physically and psychologically can be very tough. The roads seem long, the surface hard and the finish still some way off. You really have to dig deep. It's OK, you can do this.

Everyone experiences challenging moments in a marathon. It's how you respond and react to them that make or break your day. From mile 19 (30.6km) onwards, there's no room for negative thoughts. The choices you make when it hurts, to focus and keep moving, will help you believe you can achieve anything. Think beyond your limits and expectations and never stop moving forwards. When you're feeling rough and questioning if you can do it, remind yourself of how far you've come. Boost your confidence by thinking back to some of your best training runs and remember how well they went. Lock into that feeling of success and keep running. Draw on your reason for running. What's the personal reason that you going to complete the marathon? What drives you? What got you out training on cold winter nights? Whatever your reason, never give up until you reach the finish line! Try dedicating each mile in the final 5 miles (8km) to someone who has helped you on your marathon journey. As you cover the mile, run it with them in mind. Never, ever, ever give up.

Keep going, you'll reach the finish line.

THE FINISH-LINE FEELING

The finish line is such a great place. If you ever doubt human spirit and kindness, spend a few minutes watching at one. All around you there are people hugging their friends, strangers, the friends they met along the way, many are crying and some are possibly throwing up. Smaller races give you the chance to really take it all in, while at massive ones you're going to have to keep moving, when it's probably the last thing you want to do. Finish line marshals are fantastic people. They have a keen eye for people about to drop, a loud voice to remind you that you can't just stand still, and a kind 'well done' for everyone they make eye contact with. If you have enough left, make sure you thank them, too – they appreciate it. Make sure you take a moment, even if you are still being forced to move along, to take a glance back and have a moment of glory.

Finish areas can be chaotic places. It's really important here to stay calm, even though you might be feeling battered and broken. Even huge races have hiccups in this area, especially for us in the midpack who come into it at peak time. You need to do your very best to be patient in the finish area because in some races you have a long walk yet. Most finish areas won't let you cross back over the finish line again so make sure you're absolutely clear about where you are collecting your stuff from, and we mean all of it. If you are given the gift of a few minutes of waiting around that you weren't expecting, use it to stretch – it might not feel important now your race is over but it's so important to prevent you from walking like the dead tomorrow.

You're going to move through the finish area(s) on a wave of different emotions. Some finish lines will afford you a few moments to experience that rare 'I did it!' sensation, perhaps a twinge of regret and occasionally a few minutes reflecting on what might have been if only we'd done X or Y to shave a few extra seconds off.

AFTER THE RACE – RECOVERY

It's OK, and it's a good thing, to give yourself a break when race day is over. It's OK to want to stop for a bit. In fact, it's really important to do this. Your immediate recovery: stretching, changing into warm gear, eating and drinking as soon as you can, are a great start.

Just like tapering down your training, you need to allow yourself time to build back up again. Depending on your personal race calendar, the frequency of your racing, the type of race and your race priorities, recovery from races takes, and should be allocated, different amounts of time and different approaches. Recovery is a very personal thing. Race day can bring with it enormous physical and emotional stresses, following good and bad results. Every midpack runner has experienced the pride and misery of 'Tuesday legs' – the glorious struggle that means you have earned yourself a pair of legs that do not like going downstairs in a hurry, if at all.

It's very unlikely that you're going to want to nip out the day after a big race for a sharp tempo or some 800m reps on your local track. Your body feeling like it's been run over is a great signal to rest. Just like in the taper, don't let routine dictate what you do. Midpack runners are dedicated creatures of habit who often find it difficult to rest, but now is a prime opportunity to mess things up by not recovering properly. Active recovery should be your best friend. Keep moving, stand at work if you can, go for walks, and gradually prepare yourself to get back into routine with easy runs when you feel ready.

RECOVERY TIMELINE

First hour
- Collect your stuff!
- Stretch, eat, drink, find your family or friends and take that all-important medal photo.
- Change into warm gear and check on your plan for travelling home, especially if it involves public transport.

That night
- Don't start looking for what ifs. It's too early to reflect on your race too much. If it went badly, you'll be tempted to start ripping yourself apart; if it went well, you'll wish you had run it harder, or faster, or differently in some way.
- Don't start comparing yourself to others, or to a past version of yourself. Neither makes any difference to your result now.

The next day
- Empty your bag! Unpin your number, throw away anything that's going to go mouldy in your bag and get your kit wash on.
- Keep moving as much as you can and spend some time stretching and foam rolling out any sore points.

Three days later
- You're probably itching to go for a little run. Keep it very relaxed, easy, it's just there to get everything moving again.
- Start reflecting on your race lessons (see below). Write down as much as you need to.

A week later
- Refine your race lessons into what you have learned and what you can take forward to next time.
- Start picking up some of your training routine again if you feel ready. How far you run will depend on how far you raced.

AFTER THE RACE – REFLECTION

Racing represents an amazing opportunity to learn about yourself. Reflecting on your process of preparing for that race and carefully considering the outcome is a really important exercise to engage in once you've finished. But here's the really important bit: don't do it immediately after you've finished. You'll be way too emotional then and your ability to effectively reflect on, review and analyse your race can be frequently impeded by gushing emotion, deep fatigue and an inability to focus. Allow yourself to experience this immediate post-race reaction but save your more informative post-race reflection and review for two to four days after the event, when you are calmer, more considered, less instantly judgemental and more able to respond rather than simply react.

Something you can't really plan for is the mental side of recovering from a big race. Sometimes, runners in the midpack can experience a slump after a big event, when they feel a little lost and blue. If your race didn't go to plan then the slump will feel a little worse than usual, and it's OK to feel disappointed. Running is like that, especially when you aren't able to see a clear reason why it didn't work out. Sometimes you've done everything 'right' and it just wasn't your day. And that sucks. Getting over a bad experience that involved something going wrong is really valuable because you have something to work on for next time. Trying to make sense of a race when you're not sure what went wrong, though, is a little more challenging. This is another great time to engage with process. Look back over the things you got right in training, where you grew as a runner, what you learned – even down to any PBs you got along the way. Doing this is really important if you are to grow from a race, especially one that didn't go to plan. You will have made so much progress that wasn't reflected in that time on the clock. Reflection on great races is just as useful because you can draw on what made it click on the day and what made it all come together so you can do it all over again next time!

How to make sense of your race – racing lessons

Written reflection is really powerful, so make time to do this a couple of days after your race. We like to work through something like the survey below to help us make sense of the race and ultimately to grow from it. You can also find joy in doing it since it will help you to feel proud of what you achieved.

Ask yourself these important post-race questions to help your grow, learn and race again:

1. In this race, what went right for you?
   Include training, your mental prep, any logistical planning, your build-up, the days before, your start position, your pacing, your finish experience, kit, nutrition.
2. Why did these things go right?
   What did you do to facilitate this working out well? Be really specific. What else went right? (Honestly, something did, write it down.)
3. What of these things that went right are you going to continue to work on?
   List your actions for how you are going to continue to work on these things.
4. In this race, what could you have done differently?
   Again, include training, your mental preparation, logistical planning, your build-up, the days before, your start position, your pacing, your finish experience, kit, nutrition.
5. What did you love about doing the race?
   This encourages you to look for joy everywhere. Think outside the box. Did you see any great motivational signs? Was there something great in your goody bag at the end? Was there a challenging moment you're really proud to have got though?
6. What are your top five race experience takeaways?
   Read through the above and refine them into five lessons to take into your next race. Reflection in this way should throw out some key learning for you to use again.

You may also ask yourself:

- What responses did you make to events in the race that, on reflection, you could have changed?
- What drove these responses?

- What do you need to do to positively shift this response?
- How are you going to do it?
- When are you going to do it?
- Who do you need help and support from in order to facilitate these changes?

One more time?

Racing is where it's at. Despite the temptation to go again being strong, avoid making hasty decisions about something that deserves a little more planning. Take time to look at the bigger picture, try not to react too emotionally, and see how you feel in a week or two.

When you race, you can guarantee it's cultivating your running progress. It's through racing that you really get to see the fruits of your training, the results of your hard graft, the outcomes of your effort. Racing might not always look like what you want it to, happen in ways you planned, or turn out

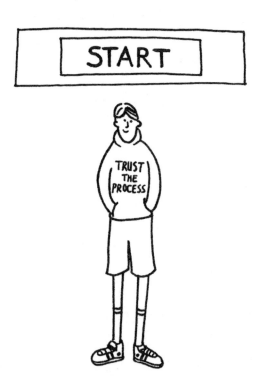

as you'd hoped, but rest assured that the race day experience shapes you as a runner, informs your ability to train and to race in the future, and impacts the ways in which you can move through the midpack. Racing nourishes your running achievements. It's made for that. It's why we do what we do as midpack runners. Searching race calendars, paying entry fees, travelling to events, getting our snappy kicks, lubing in all the places we never thought we'd lube, wearing short shorts, trying, trying again, laughing, crying, hurting, sharing, struggling, suffering, improving, celebrating. Although it might not always be striking or obvious when we initially process our race results and tell ourselves we could have done better, when the dust settles, the Tuesday legs have disappeared, the race tee has been washed, and the medal has been hung up, we realise that deep in our midpack runner self we love racing, the essence of real racing, at whatever level we participate in that brings us the greatest joy to our running. One of the most beautiful things about race day in the midpack is that, no matter how well it went, you're going to get another chance. That's why we keep throwing our hat into the racing ring. It's a rewarding roller coaster we love to ride. We get to do it again and again!

We might even still do it a little faster...

SEVEN

CONCLUSION

BRING JOY TO RUNNING

Running should bring you joy! Sometimes we know running is a hard taskmaster. Running can be your very best friend but also your worst enemy, sometimes all in the same workout! Essentially, throughout this book we've explored ways in which you might be able to discover and experience more joy in the running that you do, whatever season of running you are in, type of runner you believe you currently are or want to be in the future. Regardless of your experience, ability and self-perception, we believe that the running you do should add joy, happiness, purpose, satisfaction, contentment and fun to your life (OK, we accept you'll roll with some frustration, disappointment and despair at times!). If it doesn't, if it's stopped adding those joyful things to your life, if you want to re-ignite or even discover those things in your life then it's time to reflect on what your running means for you and how you engage with it.

Your running life is supported in pillars of training, racing, nutrition, psychology, whole body health, and all of the fundamental, complex and interrelated elements of all of these, and probably much more besides. In each chapter, we've tried to help you see a way to define and experience your running in the midpack in terms of understanding more about each element, unpacking some features of each element and then putting some things in place to help you move in the midpack – whatever that may mean for you right now and in the future.

Why you run, whoever you are and whatever your running looks like, the main thing we want you to really look back on as you reflect on this book is that of your happiness in running and as a runner. We want all of you, with your vast range of experiences, dreams, achievements, reasons and differences, to be more content as a runner. Joy in running is waiting to be found all around you in the midpack.

Joy in running. Look for it, seek it out, dive into it, rediscover it, develop it, cherish it, live with it.

Learn and practise the things that will make you more confident. Reflect on the things you're being too hard on yourself about – there are definitely going to be things for some of you, somewhere. Learn from others without too much comparison, don't be scared to ask questions and listen when people are really honest with you because they have your best interests at heart. There's joy to be found in your running if you learn some – or all – of what it takes to have mastery in running, much of which comes from trusting and learning from the process not just of your training, but in the day-to-day things that make you unique. Accept perspectives from others and learn the power of how you respond to them; involve others positively in your running life. Listen and hear how your running speaks to you. It is a powerful voice and guide to find joy.

Your identity and positioning as a 'midpack runner' might be a new thing, it might have been there for years, decades, from your childhood. It might, like it is for us, be a part of your work, part of your family, part of most of your time off work. But let's not ignore the whole of you. Let's remember, as a human we always need to have our foundations right for us to be content. We need to get great rest, have good, fulfilling relationships, know our stress buttons and how to deal with them. We need to know when to stop pressing on, when to back off, how to get the most out of our bodies by making them robust and ready to add running into the mix of what we are already asking them to do.

Throughout this book, we hope we've shown you repeatedly how your running can be such a great teacher. If you let it. If you allow it to shape and support your life, not control and dominate it. To find joy in your running you must learn how to harness its capacity to its fullness.

Look at your training by asking why? This helps frame (and reframe) what you want to achieve in your running, how you want your running to work with you, who you'd like to be as a runner. When you think you know why, just keep asking yourself why again. In about five 'whys' you'll have hit your real reason! Work towards goals that have great process along the way, teach you about yourself, allow you to get out of your comfort zone, achieve and grow. Don't be afraid to pull back, to simmer, to settle with where your running is at. You don't need to make constant furious forward progress.

Look at your training as so much more than just what you have to do. View the planning of your training as a map full of routes and micro journeys that will take you through new and exciting places full of challenges that will shape you as a midpack runner. Build things into your training that enable you to connect with your fellow midpack runners, learn from them, share learning with them, run alongside them, congratulate them, be proud that you're just like them. Trust the process of your training. Don't look too far ahead, reflect and focus on now, be honest with yourself and know what gets you fired up. Take risks where they are positive, and know when you need to back off. Think of the long game for your hopes and aspirations, but focus on the process of getting there while you train, get strong, get tired, achieve things, just miss out on things, adapt, overcome and love your running.

Bring joy to one of the core foundations of you as you experiment, learn and practise the simple joy of nutrition. Think of the fuel your body needs to do its best and learn how to use that to your advantage to fuel up your running, to get the most out of your racing. Enjoy food as much as a simple, human pleasure as well as a vital tool to make you a healthier human being and runner.

Look ahead to race day now with clear focus, preparation that may not have always gone to plan but will have given you a heap of learning experiences and growth along the way. Get ready for the buzz of the start line as you channel your nerves into amazing experiences, memories and times together with your fellow midpackers. Know your reasons why you're there. Truly celebrate the times it goes to plan, and reflect diligently when it doesn't. You have so much to learn every time and you get the chance to go again, and again, and again.

How to bring joy to running

- Always know why.
- Have strong foundations.
- Health first.
- Learn from others.
- Learn from yourself.
- Be kind to yourself, always.
- Reflect.
- Celebrate your achievements.

NOURISH RUNNING ACHIEVEMENT

How do you define your running achievements? We hope that throughout this book we've helped you to reflect on how you frame and represent your running achievements. We think understanding this is really important in midpack running. If you get it wrong, if you set your sights on outcome all the time, if your running desires are super objective, if you define yourself as a midpack runner by solely your performance-orientated running goals (not that this is a bad thing some of the time) then we think you're missing a trick to nourish your running aspirations and your running achievements. To feel nourished, you should soak up enough, you should be content without abundance, you should feel pride, self-worth, good about yourself, be confident in your place in the midpack, know that you and your running in the midpack matter. To nourish your running achievements means you feel valued and surrounded by a sense of positive, life-affirming accomplishment in your running. This may well mean a rack full of shiny finishers' medals, a bucket full of personal bests and a quilt made from your race T-shirts! But it's also about so much more than this.

Your achievements in running in the midpack can and should always look like mastering sessions, feeling fulfilled, doing your best, celebrating others, being proud and reflective of the steps you take along the way. Achievement in running in the midpack rarely looks like a race win. It's not always a PB, a course PB, a segment best, a season's best. Achievement doesn't have to be an age-graded result, a category position or a total amount of miles run each week. We value the experiential and relational elements of achievement in your running. You saw somewhere different, you ran with someone new, you paced a first-time finisher, you reflected on a race suffer-fest and it brought a smile to your face.

There's a place to frame your midpack dreams in a number on a clock. We get how important that first time, that fast time, that furthest run is. We know how important that is for you, because it is or has been for us many times over, too. We're not telling you that race times or goal distances are not important. They motivate you, they get you to do stuff, they are your call to action and they ignite competition and drive within you. Goal race times prescribe your training sessions, inspire your hard workouts, give you commonality with every other midpack runner who 'gets' what those times represent. We want you to go and achieve those results and be very proud of what it took to get you there. But truly nourishing those achievements means, again, reflecting on what it took to get them. Even when a build-up and execution of an event goes completely to plan, there will be something to learn from it. There will be things within your confidence, your foundations of you, your health, your training (especially often your training), your cross-training, your nutrition and how it all came together on race day that if you recognise them and learn how much they mattered, you can do again as you work towards the next goal.

Nourishing achievement means not being hard on yourself when it doesn't go to plan, too. There's really always something in the process that you can look back on (sometimes it takes time) and learn from. Nobody – even the speed snakes with teams around them to help them get it all right – has a simple journey to success, whatever that is to them, without a few wobbles along the way. Whether you get the time, the position, the distance or the finish line you're working towards, the process of going through it all will have its lessons.

Nourishing achievement takes time. It's not something you can really jump into overnight without being patient. You have to plant the seeds first: reflect, routine, plan. Water them: reflect, learn, ask questions. See them grow: mastery, progress, results. All of this takes time, patience and heaps of kindness to yourself.

How to nourish running achievement

- See achievement as more than always just a number on a clock or next to your name.
- Reflect.
- Be patient.
- Trust the process of training.
- Recognise and allow time for mastery to take place.

CULTIVATE YOUR PROGRESS

You will have seen throughout this book that we frequently mention bumps in the road and learning lessons. Progress in anything is rarely linear, and in running that's obviously true. Even if this were a professional endeavour there would be things that got in the way because life isn't set up to just be straightforward with no challenges. In the midpack, that's especially true. We don't expect you to build and build and build again through perfect cycles of training and superb progressive race results. We would have nothing to talk about! It's not about fearing things going wrong, either. Cultivating progress in running in the midpack looks like a ton of lessons, learning curves, achievements and setbacks. Cultivating doesn't mean perfecting. It means gently shaping and nurturing your season in the midpack so that time spent there provides you with what you want your running to be about in your life at that time, sometimes just in that moment. We know you're going to nail your workouts, get fitter, be stronger, get your head together, know how to relax, when to relax, trust people to help you and celebrate when it all comes together.

Cultivating progress doesn't mean sticking religiously to rigid structures, enforced fancy plans, or controlled performance pathways. Looking after yourself and your running happens with healthy, consistent routines, by being in control of your running rather than allowing it to control you, by understanding why you are motivated by certain things and how these things can be built into your life in such a way that your running moves in the direction that you want it to. Cultivating progress means knowing what turns you off, too. It means understanding dysfunction in your running, having the courage to call yourself out (even when you've been doing something that way for a very long time) and the conviction to shift direction, respond with care, to be visionary and creative with what you want your running to look like and to bravely point yourself that way. We hope this book has helped you to appropriately see, plan and realise ways to grow as you move towards aspirations, challenges, targets and changes in your midpack running.

How to cultivate your progress

- Accept, but don't expect, difficult times.
- Know what made a workout or a race great.
- Develop healthy routines.
- Link process and progress together.
- Monitor and measure your progress regularly, but know that it won't always be in a straight line or upwards curve (and definitely don't obsess about it!).
- Be patient. Deep change and real progress take time but are worth the wait.
- Value and trust in your relationships.

Sometimes in life, really and completely unexpected things happen. Running is exactly the same. Your build-up might go spectacularly well, you could be hitting every workout, feeling amazing. You might have your head together, foundations strong, focus absolutely nailed and it might just not happen for you. Races get cancelled for a number of reasons, the rug pulled out from under you and potentially that focus and end goal taken out of your hands and out of your control. If you have understood this book as we intend it, you will be in a good position to know how to respond to even the most challenging of midpack scenarios with purpose.

We wrote this book in 2020, as we were hit by a global pandemic, the scale of which we had never seen before. For the first time in our memory as runners, we could no longer run with our friends, or train in the same ways we had done up until now. We had no tangible end goals. Races everywhere were cancelled. Our calendars were empty and we were forced to run for different reasons, with different focus and often in different places. The coronavirus pandemic is an extreme example of things happening beyond our control, but it's relevant because everyone reading this book will have made their own adjustments to running, and they will remember how that felt. This book should help you see opportunity. We know that opportunity emerges sometimes when you least expect it. We'd urge you to step back sometimes, notice and be open to opportunity in the midpack. It might not look like what you expect. When you're used to pushing to the front, give yourself permission and celebrate taking your foot off the gas, experience your running differently. When you're used to inhabiting a midpack of comfort and control we'd urge you to explore discomfort, to push yourself in different ways, to ask new and exciting things from yourself and from your running. We hope, in a small way, this book gives you a toolkit that prepares you to respond better, flex through difficult or unexpected changes that inevitably come with being the runner you really want to be.

We want this to be a book that encourages you to create great memories of your running that turn into even better stories. Whatever season you're in as a runner, we want you to create stories you can tell again and again when you're in the next season. Telling stories about the time this happened is better than just telling stories about the time ran. Weave together experiences and outcomes that nourish achievement, cultivate progress and bring joy to your running.

That's where the best stories happen.

FINAL THOUGHTS

In the time it has taken us to write *Running in the Midpack*, I have run two marathons, I've felt the heartbreak of just missing out on target times I'd poured months of work into, had unexpected race results, run amazing long runs with friends, got injured, explored new places, made mistakes with nutrition, overtrained, changed training strategies. I have listened, learned, not listened, learned more. I've run in appalling weather, along beaches in the summer, and throughout winter in the dark. I have done sessions that I thought were too easy, then too hard, probably consulted my watch too many times, spent a lot of money on race entry and kit. I've heard the roar of the crowds in big city races, I have ended up on my own adrift of the pack in the middle of nowhere. In short, I've done everything many of you have done many times over. The process of writing the book, thinking about what makes us as midpack runners move and passionately care about our running made me look into myself as a runner, too.

We really wanted you to see that the midpack is for everyone, and that fast or slow are relative terms because regardless of outcome, you're working hard for it. You invest your time in your running and that is enough for us. The midpack is a great place because we always have time to grow and change as we change and learn as runners, as friends, as humans. Coaching midpack runners is joyful and ever-changing but many ask the same things of us, and that's where the idea for this book came. We hope that if you've been running for many years, taken a step back from faster running into the midpack, dusted off your trainers after a break away from running, or just always belonged there, that you've been able to find something in this book to relate to. It excites me to think that someone somewhere might unlock something special in their running that they'd forgotten about or never tried, that might make them happier, calmer, more organised, less stressed, more confident midpack runners.

It really is all about process.

We are pouring our hearts into a pursuit that is always measurable and comparable to others and that's why it can just feel a bit exposing and messy. But truly focusing on the process is where the joy in running is waiting to be found or rediscovered. It's about growing through the experiences you have along the way and valuing each and every one of them. Running is a blessing and reflecting on the process of doing it is a powerful thing.

I'll see you in the midpack.

Anji Andrews

***

What a run! I once tried to run the entire length of the South West Coast Path in 20 days. It's 630 miles (1014km) from Minehead to Poole with a colossal elevation profile and too many small steps up and down than I can remember. I didn't finish it. After a 260-mile (418km), seven-day, 17,000m (56,000ft) elevation week I ended up at Land's End, reasonably broken. Spending 10 hours on the trails every day, with average daily speeds of 2–3mph (3.2–4.8kph), that path really is my nemesis. It's a place in running that is also hugely important to me. Despite not being able to complete the route (I stopped at day 15 for all sorts of complicated reasons), I learned so much.

I've been running for more than 40 years and so my journey in the 'midpack' has been informed by the power of running breathing into my life almost every day. I certainly did not regard 'not finishing the SWCP' as a failure. In fact, it was a privilege to experience it. And it was less painful than that fall on the cinder track aged nine in the Yeovil district schools' athletics championships, and being picked up, crying my heart out, by my mum!

Sharing the journey with my wife of her experiences at the pointy end of the sharpest midpack in the world allowed me to piggyback on the running lives of the some of the fastest runners in world. Running with African friends, with parkrun friends, with nervous London Marathon first-time friends, running with a 5-minute-miler and a 25-minute-miler is a privilege. Talking about running every week on 'Marathon Talk' has opened my eyes to the stories of amazing runners and the incredible running communities they live in. I'm shown time and time again that running literally does saves lives. It saves people from breakdown, from addiction, from others, from themselves. Running is a safe, trusted, certain, secure, happy, exciting, challenging, adventurous, rewarding, joyful, cultivating, nourishing place to live.

And the midpack is it's beating heart. And you're right there in the middle of it. Enjoy every run.

Martin Yelling

Acknowledgements

Our thanks

Many thanks to our contributors Mimi Anderson, Anita Bean, Dr Georgie Bruinvels, Paul Hobrough, Steve Ingham, Prof Andy Lane, Steve Magness, Dr Simon Marshall, Colin McCourt, Renee McGregor, Dr Josie Perry, Dr Jess Piasecki, Dan Robinson and Paul Tonkinson. You all gave so much time and expertise and we truly appreciate it.

Thank you Ryan Hall for saying it so well and allowing us to use your words.

To Matt Lowing at Bloomsbury for believing in an idea and making it a reality. You have been supportive, kind and creative throughout the process of writing this book and we couldn't have done this without your vision.

Thank you to our brilliant editor Holly Jarrald for supporting the book during the important final stages.

Thank you to everyone who gave the time to have conversations about what makes midpack runners who they are. To Adam Jones, Evan Davies, Stephanie Knox, Neale Bulbeck, Emma Kovaleski, Michael Briggs, Sarah Dudgeon, Phil Connor, Caroline Ames, Charlotte Proud and Kevin Jeffress.

To the Marathon Talk family and community who inspire, motivate and delight us with relentless positivity. Thank you.

Anji's thanks

Writing *Running in the Midpack* came in phases for us. Things moved very quickly in the initial idea and planning for the book but writing, like running, came in seasons. The process was nothing like I expected, in fact it was far more joyful and I learned a great deal about myself as a runner as I wrote about others. It was cathartic to research and write about the things that had brought me so much happiness and connection in running. I think this book made me more reflective as a runner and it made me better.

I have to start by thanking Martin for his invaluable partnership in writing this book. As a creator, he has been fun, he's made me cry with laughter ('You don't have to get your monk on'). As a mentor he's made me think, challenge myself and pushed me to write in a different way. As a friend, he's made me have the difficult conversations some of you will have had in your head as you read the book. He is always dependable at any time of the day or night. We've written together, remotely, online, over video call, via long emails, at all times of day. We have had our best creative ideas running side by side in Dorset and in France, we've had days sitting in cafes drinking endless cups of what he would say was too-posh coffee. We had times changing each other's writing online before the other person even finished, and we still remained friends. We have just had to trust the process. Thank you for everything Martin.

Thank you to my husband Paul for the patience it's taken to answer my many many questions of him as the classic front of the midpack runner and for all the times he's had to listen to my reading aloud of sections that just didn't sound right. You run faster and further than I could dream of, but it's your kindness and beautiful heart that inspires me the most. We have so many more miles and adventures ahead together. Take my hand, and run.

To my family: Mam, Lee, Kerri and Sam. You inspire me and make me who I am, and I love you.

Thank you Ruby, Beau, Sonny and Liz Yelling for everything it's taken to accommodate this project into your life, and at times me into your home. Liz, you have always inspired me as an incredible athlete and a beautiful human being and you continue to do so.

My best friends Jen, Guy and David, none of you are runners and still remain positive and supportive about whatever crazy challenge I am engrossed in including this one. You have known me as non runner, runner and now writer and you've supported me no matter what. I love you. 'When I'm with you, I'm standing with an army.'

Thank you to Dan Robinson, an outstanding coach and physiologist who gave me so much time and so many resources. I'm grateful for the friendship you showed me throughout writing this book.

Thanks to Luke for his brilliant coaching input, despite usually taking three working days to answer a text.

Thank you to Sally for running the most and the best miles with me. We have had the best experiences together and many miles ahead ... get the itinerary ready!

Thank you to Phil Hewitt for giving me my first experience of writing for a book about running. I am grateful for the friendship, advice and opportunity you have brought my way.

Thank you Phil Thomas, an inspiring midpack runner, excellent secret keeper and Best Man.

To everyone I have run with in the midpack as a leader, as a fellow parkrunner, as your coach, in races, in clubs. Thank you for the enthusiasm, the company, the connections and the fun that made me want to write this book for you.

In memory of a beautiful person and popular midpack runner, Marcus Gynn. You were somebody who made everybody feel like somebody.

Martin's thanks

Learning to do anything is about the people who teach and guide you to do it. People who we learn from teach us the things we live by. There have been, and continue to be, many amazing teachers in my life who have walked and run with me, picked me up when I've fallen down, given me confidence to keep going, helped me realise aspirations and shared the glorious run at life we're privileged to be on together.

This book is a thanks to all of them.

Thank you to my wife, Liz and children, Ruby, Sonny and Beau for smiling through the late hours and early mornings of phone calls, tapping on the laptop, and out-loud mind-wanders. Liz is one of those amazing teachers who through gentle kindness, compassion, humility and love allows me to be creative, curious, disappointed and ambitious. She is my forever life and running partner and her wisdom, strength, resilience and patience inspires me every day.

Thanks to all of the running coaches that have been a part of my life and shaped my own experiences and understandings of what it means to run and to be a runner.

Thanks to all of the runners out there I've learned so much from and had the pleasure of coaching on their own personal running journeys. Every runner I've worked with teaches me something new about my own running through their own experiences of running. Every runner I've run with, thank you.

Thanks to the amazing Marathon Talk running community and my podcasting brother Tom Williams. So much running chat over the years.

Thank you to my co-author Anji. Someone who seeks to understand, who goes the extra mile, who suffered my ramblings and waffle and was prepared to work together to laugh our way through writing a book about running.

Thanks to my Mum for a love of words.

* * *

This book is for you, the reader and runner, to perhaps look at your running differently, to truly see what you love about being a runner and to understand how to use that to teach yourself how to be the kind of runner you'd like to be.

Index